WHY EXERCISE?

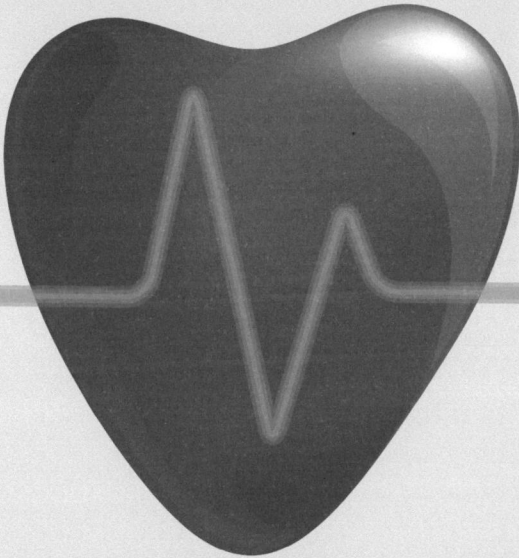

THE FACTS FOR A HEALTHY LIFESTYLE

ANTHONY AURELIUS

Printed and Published in the United Kingdom by

Real World Publishing Ltd.

108 Wick Street
Littlehampton
West Sussex
United Kingdom
BN17 7JS

Tel. 0845 450 6605
www.rwpgroup.com

Book Cover Design by Luke Metcalfe at RWP

Photo by Michael Chevis
www.michaelchevis.com

First Edition

ISBN 978-0-9557588-0-5

"Having known Anthony for many years now I can honestly say that he brings to this book a great dedication, integrity and love, and is an absolute living example of what he teaches."

"This book really gets to the heart of the matter in a direct and concise way, that is not only dynamic and intuitive but also demonstrates the skills that the author has, representing a huge amount of study, training, research and dedication."

"Covering all of the main aspects and benefits of exercise this powerful book is a must read for anyone who wants to increase their overall well-being in life."

Gerard Donovan, Founder of Noble Manhattan Coaching Ltd, CEO of The European Coaching Institute

"Clear, concise and to the point, Anthony cuts through the maze of 21st century hyperbole and spin with a strong attack on today's sedentary lifestyle."

"Fully referenced, this 'manual for fitness' is a must read for everyone, from a person thinking of taking their first steps on the road to fitness, to the 'exercise guru' who wants the details about the need for exercise at their fingertips."

"Everyone with an interest in training NEEDS this book ...WHY EXERCISE?...This is the book that explains it!"

Pete Ryan Dip, ISSA CFT SPN www.veganbodybuilding.org

"I have spent 15 years working as a top Personal Trainer and Nutritionist to the general public at large, and also many celebrities. I have been privileged enough to know Anthony Aurelius for ten years. It is truly rare to meet someone with Anthony's integrity, skill and passion. I can honestly say that he is an inspiration to everyone he comes into contact with. He is a true pioneer and I am honoured to of worked and trained with him."

Justin House, YMCA PT, Stars of Tomorrow Champion O2

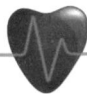

"Exercise is essential for all of the reasons stated in Anthony's book, reading this book will save you endless hours of research. Putting it to good use will enhance and extend your life. I have known Anthony for 10 years and his dedication and belief in ultimate health has never weakened. This book will motivate, shock and inspire you. This book will educate many and inspire them to improve their lives and those of the ones they love."

Heather Mills McCartney

"If you ever have to question why you have to exercise, this book is the answer!"

"There are no ifs or buts, we all have to exercise if we value our lives. The research says it all."

"I would suggest you leave this out on your coffee table and you might save someone's life or at least give them a chance to save their own, (and become happier in the bargain)."

Petra Tanner, Specialist Physiotherapist, The Oving Clinic for Sports and Exercise Medicine

"As a former bodybuilding champion and success coach, health and wellness has been my life for the past 25 years, and I've read hundreds of books on the subject."

"Anthony is a product of what he teaches. This latest book will really put the WHY into your action plan, it will focus your efforts on Prevention. We know you can choose to forget your health however your health won't forget you, so take action today."

Marc Raymond, NABBA Bodybuilding Champion, FITPRO Personal Trainer, BAWLA Coach, Clinical Nutritionist

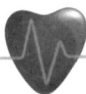

About the Author

Anthony Aurelius, as well as being known in the media, is also the International Spokesperson for Choi Kwang Do Martial Art International www.choikwangdo.com. Choi Kwang Do is a peaceful, non-violent but practical martial art that has been designed for character development, self-defence and optimum health and fitness. Anthony has trained with the National Academy of Sports Medicine www.nasm.org and Braingym www.braingym.com. He is also a trained counsellor, a professionally qualified coach with the European Coaching Institute www.europeancoachinginstitute.org and a trained Emotional Freedom Technique (EFT) Practitioner, www.emofree.com. Anthony has over twenty-five years of experience of teaching martial arts and fitness around the world to both groups and individuals.

Anthony still trains a number of high-profile clients around the world who are serious about valuing their health. He also directs a company, Warrior Challenge Events www.warriorchallenge-events.co.uk that runs fun, unique and exciting team building days that are a good foundation toward improving fitness, health and performance long-term.

Anthony is Vegan, so he doesn't use animal products of any kind and he doesn't eat meat, eggs, fish or diary. This he says, "is better for the animals, the environment, and my health". Although he has used evidence from scientific studies conducted in this book on mice and rats, these experiments have happened, but he does not support testing on animals.

If you are looking to work one-to-one with Anthony as a Personal Trainer, or in any capacity, please get in touch with his agent, Karin Ridgers at MAD Promotions "For people who are Making A Difference' within UK office hours on Tel. +44 (0) 7970 732668 or via Email. info@mad-promotions.com

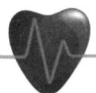

I dedicate this book to the one I love.

You are the most beautiful woman
in the world.

Always & Forever...
Until my heart leaves this earth...
And my body dies...
I will be here to help you...

My Deep Love for you will exist
Always...

I Promise You.

Anthony Aurelius

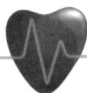

CONTENTS

Foreword 8-9

Introduction 10-11

1. Why Exercise? To Prevent Disease 12-24

2. Aerobic Training for Optimum Health....................................25-32

3. Anaerobic Training for Optimum Health 33-38

4. Resistance Training for Optimum Health.................................39-48

5. Stretching/Flexibility Training for Optimum Health...................49-57

6. To Prevent or Reverse Weight Gain or Obesity.........................58-66

7. To Prevent Cardiovascular Disease 67-79

8. To Prevent Cancer..80-90

9. To Prevent or Reverse Depression 91-99

10. To Prevent or Reverse Diabetes 100-108

11. To Prevent or Reverse Arthritis...109-116

12. To Prevent or Reverse Osteoporosis...................................117-125

13. To Prevent or Reduce Back Pain 126-130

14. To Prevent Alzheimer's Disease 131-136

15. To Prevent Parkinson's Disease 137-141

16. To Prevent Multiple Sclerosis...142-147

17. To Ensure Optimum Health & Longevity.............................148-157

18. To Positively Influence Children 158-160

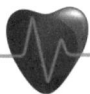

FOREWORD

Intuitively we all know exercise is good, maybe even essential. Each January 1st many of us start off with renewed resolve and an ambitious plan. But slowly the demands of everyday living take over, always for a good reason. Or so we think.

Why such repeated failure? Because intuition and good intentions are not enough. We need a more soundly based rational belief and then a programme which is practical and pragmatic. Anthony Aurelius gives us both in this systemic approach to exercise.

For years I have been diligent about aerobic training. I enjoy running even to the extent of accepting the pain of several marathons. But only latterly, when exercising with Anthony, have I understood the importance of anaerobic and resistance training and the role of stretching to maintain flexibility. Each has its part, in a programme of fitness for life.

And it literally is for life – extending it and enhancing its quality. While exercise in itself will not ensure we avoid ailments and sickness, in combination with sensible living, it makes us a tougher nut to crack.

Anthony brings the rationale reasoning together forcefully and convincingly. He shows us how exercise impacts on every aspect of our living. Then he shows us how to put our new found conviction into action.

I built my career with one of the world's most successful multinational companies for 37 years. I was lucky enough to be CEO for 8 years. My

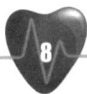

job and those of my colleagues were demanding, stressful and at times physically exhausting. I saw at first hand the importance of physical fitness to mental agility and effective leadership. I came to understand that one of the most important responsibilities of the leader is to ensure that the team care for their health and fitness.

If you are truly interested in a longer and more active life, and having fun, read this book and act on its advice. Of course if you are not interested then you are making a choice probably to the detriment of your health and longevity.

Niall W A FitzGerald KBE

Chairman Reuters PLC

Chairman International Business Council

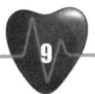

Introduction

I decided to publish this book after reading so many fascinating scientific studies that were clearly illustrating the benefits of exercise - I myself was shocked. It was at this time that I honestly felt that more people really needed to read the material that I was finding so interesting, and not just a select few. Hence, I put this book together.

Over the years I have read countless exercise books with glossy photos of models performing exercises with 'perfect bodies' and with 'perfect technique'. Indeed, most of the people I train, or have trained over the years have wanted to work with me as a personal trainer for cosmetic reasons, at first anyway. Furthermore, the majority of people that I talk to still believe that exercise is just done to look good, and that it has little to do with health. **This perspective needs to change because exercise really is an essential component of a healthy lifestyle, along with optimum nutrition and human love.**

Upon passing the content of this book (before going to print) to a wonderful friend of mine for his feedback, Matthew, (who is also a client who I train weekly, his whole family actually too) I also gave a few chapters to his fourteen-year-old daughter to read. After reading these chapters she returned them to me and said, 'frightening'.

I have mixed feelings about Suzanna's reaction. My goal in publishing this book has definitely not been to frighten anyone. My deep hope is that it will motivate more people to exercise than ever before, but not once or twice a week, one month on, one month off - but 5-6 days a week for life!

Please take responsibility for your health and exercise regularly, especially if you are a mother or a father, grandmother or grandfather: your life is important not just to yourself but to your children and/or your grandchildren, and also others around you who love you dearly.

Nothing is more important than your health. Exercise for life!

Wholeheartedly,

Anthony Aurelius

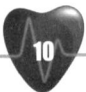

The definition of insanity:

*to keep doing the same things
and expect different results.*

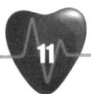

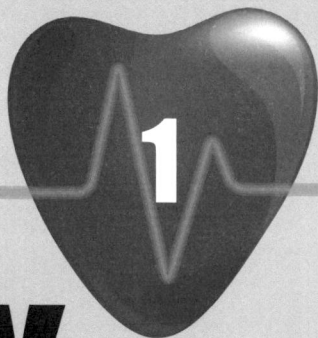

WHY
EXERCISE?
To Prevent Disease

1

Why Exercise? - To Prevent Disease

Degenerative Diseases

Throughout our lifetime, survival requires that we remain robust and adaptable. We must be able to live through a wide range of experiences and environments. Because life can expose us to minor and more serious degenerative diseases, our aim should be to remain in optimum health.

Degenerative diseases can develop over a period of time, with the symptoms and signs becoming progressively worse. This can lead to the affected person's life becoming increasingly difficult. Often, this lifestyle change is irreversible once disease sets in.

Although any part of the body can be involved, three systems in particular are prone to debilitating degenerative diseases - the nervous system, the muscular system, and the skeletal system.

Diseases that can be prevented include

- Obesity
- Cardiovascular Disease (CVD)
- Cancer
- Depression
- Diabetes
- Arthritis
- Osteoporosis
- Back Pain
- Alzheimer's Disease
- Parkinson's Disease
- Multiple Sclerosis

Chronic Diseases are Epidemic

Recent data from the Centres for Disease Control document that cardiovascular diseases, various forms of cancer, and diabetes combine to make up 70% of all deaths in the western world. [1] Additionally, overweight and obesity [as defined by a body mass index (BMI) are at epidemic levels. [2, 3] Diabetes mellitus (once known as adult-onset diabetes), and metabolic syndrome are now common in children. [4]

Chronic diseases present an enormous burden to society by increasing medical costs and human suffering. [5] **Recent data estimates that physical inactivity and poor diet will soon rank as the leading causes of death in the western world**. [6] This may even be an underestimate, given that it reflects deaths attributable only to those with obesity, when, in fact, physical inactivity and inappropriate diet impact mortality at any BMI. [7]

Although these health problems (CVD, diabetes, etc.) have been virtually non-existent in underdeveloped countries, they are now on the rise everywhere as people change their diets and become more sedentary. [8] Physical activity and diet are effective interventions for what leading researchers have coined, "the war on chronic disease." [9, 10] Clearly, there is overwhelming evidence linking most chronic diseases seen in the world today to physical inactivity and inappropriate dietary consumption.

J Appl. Physiol. 98: 3-30, 2005
Effects of Exercise and Diet on Chronic Disease

Currently, modern chronic diseases, including cardiovascular diseases, Type 2 diabetes, metabolic syndrome and cancer are the leading killers in Westernised society. These diseases are also increasingly rampant in developing nations. In fact, obesity, diabetes, and hypertension are now even commonplace in children.

However, there are solutions to this epidemic of metabolic disease that is inundating today's societies worldwide: exercise and diet. Overwhelming evidence from a variety of sources links most prevalent chronic diseases to physical inactivity and an inappropriate diet.

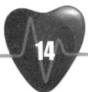

Adaptations to Exercise

The Principle of Adaptation (S.A.I.D)

The S.A.I.D principle states that whatever specific physical exercise programme/physical activity we choose to perform, our bodies will adapt specifically to the imposed demands of this particular activity.

S = Specific
A = Adaptation
I = Imposed
D = Demands

A carefully designed exercise programme can therefore have a tremendous impact on the outcome of the practitioner.

Order of Adaptation

1. LOCAL
2. CENTRAL
3. PSYCHOLOGICAL

This order of adaptation occurs until demands cease to increase. Both central and local adaptations are critical to improve the resilience and health of an individual.

Local adaptations > Cellular change
(i.e. structure, vascular, chemical and mechanical efficiency)

Central adaptation > Circulatory system, immune system, capillary density

Psychological Adaptation > Improved Mental Attitude

Levels of Exercise

Humans living today have inherited a genome that was programmed for daily physical activity and a high-fibre diet. [11] Nevertheless, most people today have the perception that genes cause chronic disease. However, more and more people are beginning to recognise they need to exercise, and eat a healthy, balanced diet.

An Introduction to Genes

Cells

The human cell is the smallest functional body unit capable of life processes. It is the basic living unit of all organisms. All organisms are made up of one or more cells e.g. liver cells, skin cells, muscle cells, brain cells, bone cells, etc.

The human body is made up of many systems that interact with each other, but bones, muscles, blood, skin, nerves and other tissues are, in reality, just millions to billions of connected cells.

The nucleus of each cell contains 46 chromosomes (23 pairs). These chromosomes are coiled molecules of DNA. Genes are tiny regions of DNA that dictate cell activity.

Genes

The super-coiled DNA structure simply consists of four different chemicals that are arranged in pairs that interlock. These four chemicals are held together between two lines, (which are made up of sugar-phosphate molecules).

Scientists refer to the 4 chemicals as the base, or 4 bases. The 4 bases are as follows:

T – Thymine, A – Adenine, C – Cytosine, G – Guanine

The structure of the gene dictates the function. If the gene loses its base structure, it will not function properly. All disease is now known to be, at its most fundamental level, a gene mutation. This means that the gene loses its base sequence and therefore cannot function properly.

J Appl Physiol 200:019265, 2002

Exercise and gene expression: physiological regulation of the human genome through physical activity.

The authors of this study proposed that gene regulation was selected during an era of obligatory physical activity, as the survival of our late (50,000-10,000 BC) ancestors depended on hunting and gathering. A sedentary lifestyle in such an environment probably meant elimination of that individual organism.

Living environments today are predominantly sedentary, resulting in abnormal gene expression, which in turn manifests itself as disease.

The authors of this study contend that the current scientific evidence supports the notion that disruptions in cellular homeostasis are diminished in magnitude within physically active individuals. This disruption level is low compared with sedentary individuals due to the natural selection of gene expression that supports the physically active lifestyle displayed by our ancestors. They speculate that genes evolved with the expectation of requiring a certain threshold of physical activity for normal physiologic gene expression, and thus habitual exercise in sedentary cultures restores perturbed homeostatic mechanisms towards the normal physiological range of Homo Sapiens.

Research is confirming that physical activity is essential for gene regulation and health. Too much exercise, (overtraining) on the other hand, can suppress gene regulation.

The Overtraining Syndrome

Sedentary lifestyles are not the only problems that arise from this prehistory gene selection. In addition, excessive, competitive or hard training can lead to the overtraining syndrome. This syndrome can be

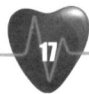

defined as a state of prolonged fatigue and underperformance caused by hard training and competition. For athletes, the stress of competition and selection pressures may also contribute to prolonged fatigue. High intensity sports training is for the purpose of winning, it has little to do with health.

High-Intensity Sports/Athletic Training

Recent research conducted by the Department of Medicine, St. George's Hospital Medical School, London, suggests that although moderate exercise is good for the immune system, the demanding training programmes of many top athletes may suppress the immune system and thereby increase susceptibility to illness and disease. A number of top athletes have suffered from unusual infections normally associated with immune deficiency, and immune abnormalities have been demonstrated in resting samples from top athletes.

Studies from several exercise laboratories have shown that, after a single exhausting exercise session, there is temporary immune depression. This marked depression is accompanied by significant changes in numbers and functional capacities of lymphocytes. These changes, which last up to several hours, are seen in both athletes and untrained individuals. In several studies in the United States, students who were very active in sports have been shown to be more susceptible to infections than their less-active colleagues. Exercising hard can increase the severity of illness.

Exercise stress needs to be managed. Research indicates that both male and female competitive athletes and ballet dancers who subject themselves to greater levels of physical demands have negative physiological outcomes. These athletes perform hard in order to win over many years. As a result, they produce fewer sperm or egg cells and live shorter lives.

Oxidative Stress – The Free-Radical

Molecules are made of atoms bonded together. This bonding process is done by sharing electrons. When two atoms join, their electrons pair up

to make a stable molecule. When an oxygen molecule splits, it becomes unstable because of the loss of electrons that were originally paired in the molecule. This is called a free radical, and is oxidative stress. These molecules can damage cells by a process called oxidation, which is like the "rusting" of a human cell.

Makoto Kuro-o, Assistant Professor of Pathology at the University of Texas Southwestern Medical Center, said, "**Increased longevity is always associated with increased resistance to oxidative stress**. Oxidative stress causes the accumulation of oxidative damage to important biological macromolecules: lipids, proteins and DNA. This results in functional deterioration of the cell."

Epigenetics

"Epigenetics" is a new emerging science. It is proving that **what we eat – and how we live and love – alters the way our genes behave**.

Growing scientific evidence is emerging to support the importance of the emerging field of epigenetics. A report from Duke University Medical Centre (DUMC) recently covered some startling scientific discoveries.

Growing data is proving the way environmental stress (even in embryonic or fetal development) can increase an individual's susceptibility to a host of diseases and behavioural responses in life.

Randy Jirtle, Ph.D., a genetics researcher in Duke's Department of Radiation Oncology, said, "We can no longer argue whether genes or environment has a greater impact on our health and development, because both are inextricably linked."

In addition, Fred Tyson, Ph.D. at the National Institute of Environmental Health Sciences (NIEHS), said, "Each nutrient, each interaction, each experience can manifest itself through biochemical changes that ultimately dictate gene expression, whether at birth or 40 years down the road."

Epigenetics is proving how important our environment and our lifestyle habits are for our long-term health. In a huge number of scientific studies, nutritious eating habits, drinking an adequate amount of water throughout the day, and participation in low to moderate levels of exercise is proving

essential to long-term health and wellness.

Loving and nurturing relationships of support and encouragement are also essential for our health and happiness. So, the stress related to highly competitive sports or business environments may be extremely hazardous to health.

R. Jirtle stated that bad genes can sadly be passed down from one generation to the next. But he went on to detail the good news: they are reversible; genes can potentially change with nutrients and enriched experiences.

The fact that science has now confirmed that gene behaviour is not hereditary, and the fact that genes are far more malleable than we once believed could explain the dramatic rise in obesity, cancer, heart disease, diabetes and other chronic diseases in prosperous nations. Indeed, the inhabitants of prosperous, "quick fix" nations tend to eat poor diets and live computer-based, car driving, sedentary lifestyles.

"**The more that is learned about genes, the less DNA looks like it is hereditary**", Moshe Szyf, an epigeneticist at Canada's McGill University, declared.

Genes can change according to an individual's environment. It's part of the reason why "identical" twins can be so different. In a report, Szyf said that people need to address the environmental aspects of health.

"Epigenetics is one of the fastest-moving areas of science, period", said Melanie Ehrlich, a Tulane University epigeneticist whose laboratory linked cancer to lifestyle in 1983.

In the past two decades – and especially over the last couple of years – research has shown that disease can change in response to environment and lifestyle habits.

Disease or bad habits?

Worldwide, scientists are now confirming that chronic degenerative disease is related to lifestyle or environmental stress. Continual stress or "bad lifestyle habits" cause the gene to mutate, to lose its base structure. Once the gene loses its base structure, it loses the ability to function properly.

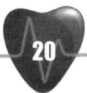

Negative factors can damage cells and genes.

These factors include

- Stress
- Poor diet
- Smoking
- Drinking
- Pollution
- Chemicals
- Radiation
- **A lack of (or too much) physical exercise**
- Negative thought and negative emotions

Lifestyle Changes can Reverse Disease Progress

For over a hundred years, groups have researched the causes of chronic diseases, such as CVD. [12] Consequently, the search for therapies that can prevent and reverse existing disease has been conducted over this same time period. Early studies focused on cholesterol and saturated fat and their relation to CVD, whereas more recent studies have progressed to investigate diabetes, hypertension, cancer, and metabolic syndrome. This has been emphasised in a recent report from the World Health Organization (WHO). [8]

Diet has been known for years to play a key role as a risk factor for chronic diseases. Traditional, largely plant-based diets have been replaced by high-fat, energy-dense diets with a substantial content of animal foods. However, though diet is critical to prevention, it is just one risk factor. **Physical exercise is now being recognized as not optional, but essential for living a long and healthy life**.

There is overwhelming evidence that diet, smoking, alcohol, and physical inactivity are important determinants of CVD and other chronic disorders and that modifying these environmental influences can significantly impact the incidence of chronic disease. Evidence over the past 20 years from a variety of sources, including epidemiological and

intervention studies, has documented that good lifestyle choices can mitigate the progression of chronic disease. Furthermore, **evidence is compiling to point out that healthy lifestyle changes can, in fact, reverse existing disease**.

With respect to physical activity, **recent studies have highlighted the importance of regular physical activity in decreasing the risk of chronic disease**, [13, 14] emphasising that humans have evolved to be active.

Also, **in 2002, the Institute of Medicine recommended one hour of moderate physical activity daily**, "to accrue additional, weight-independent health benefits." This recommendation was supported by the WHO report. According to research, this daily activity should include both aerobic and resistance exercise. [9, 15, 8, 16, 17]

Given the ineffectiveness of popular weight-loss diets, adoption of a healthy lifestyle is more appropriate for winning the war against chronic disease. [18] **There is overwhelming scientific evidence supporting the value of daily exercise** and a diet that focuses on the consumption of whole grains, fruits, and vegetables. **This evidence shows that these lifestyle choices can prevent and treat the major diseases seen in the industrialised countries today**.

Evidence proves that one hour of daily physical activity should be performed in combination with the consumption of a natural food diet. This diet of course should be high in fibre-containing fruits, vegetables, and whole grains, and naturally low in fat. The diet should also contain abundant amounts of vitamins, minerals, and phytochemicals. By combining this type of diet with physical activity, the vast majority of chronic disease may be prevented.

In summary:

- **Modern life is dangerous to your health! We are all programmed by nature to live physically active lives. If we ignore this fact, our bodies become genetically unbalanced, opening the door to chronic disease.**

- **Lack of exercise and poor eating habits will soon be the leading cause of death in the western world.**

- **However, YOU can reverse this trend. Correct, regular exercise,**

combined with an improved diet, can keep you healthier for longer …
and even help reverse any existing heath problems. It's never too late
to start.

Chapter References

1. Arias E, Anderson RN, Kung HC, Murphy SL, and Kochanek KD. Deaths: final data for 2001. Natl Vital Stat Rep 52: 1–115, 2003.

2. Flegal KM, Carroll MD, Kuczmarski RJ, and Johnson CL. Overweight and obesity in the United States: prevalence and trends, 1960–1994. Int J Obes Relat Metab Disord 22: 39–47, 1998.

3. Mokdad AH, Bowman BA, Ford ES, Vinicor F, Marks JS, and Koplan JP. The continuing epidemics of obesity and diabetes in the United States. JAMA 286: 1195–1200, 2001.

4. Troiano RP and Flegal KM. Overweight children and adolescents: description, epidemiology, and demographics. Pediatrics 101: 497–504, 1998.

5. Hoffman C, Rice D, and Sung HY. Persons with chronic conditions. Their prevalence and costs. JAMA 276: 1473–1479, 1996.

6. Mokdad AH, Marks JS, Stroup DF, and Gerberding JL. Actual causes of death in the United States, 2000. JAMA 291: 1238–1245, 2004.

7. Blair SN, Kohl HW 3rd, Barlow CE, Paffenbarger RS Jr, Gibbons LW, and Macera CA. Changes in physical fitness and all-cause mortality. A prospective study of healthy and unhealthy men. JAMA 273: 1093–1098, 1995.

8. Diet, nutrition, and the prevention of chronic diseases. World Health Organ Tech Rep Ser 916: i–viii, 1–149, 2003.

9. Booth FW, Chakravarthy MV, Gordon SE, and Spangenburg EE. Waging war on physical inactivity: using modern molecular ammunition against an ancient enemy. J Appl Physiol 93: 3–30, 2002.

10. Booth FW, Gordon SE, Carlson CJ, and Hamilton MT. Waging war on modern chronic diseases: primary prevention through exercise biology. J Appl Physiol 88: 774–787, 2000.

11. Eaton SB and Konner M. Paleolithic nutrition. A consideration of its nature and current implications. N Engl J Med 312: 283–289, 1985.

12. Connor WE. Diet-heart research in the first part of the 20th century. Acta Cardiol 54: 135–139, 1999.

13. Blair SN, Kohl HW 3rd, Paffenbarger RS Jr, Clark DG, Cooper KH, and Gibbons LW. Physical fitness and all-cause mortality. A prospective study of healthy men and women. JAMA 262: 2395–2401, 1989.

14. Booth FW, Chakravarthy MV, and Spangenburg EE. Exercise and gene expression: physiological regulation of the human genome through physical

activity. J Physiol 543: 399–411, 2002.

15. Dietary Reference Intakes for Energy, Carbohydrate, Fiber, Fat, Fatty Acids, Cholesterol, Protein, and Amino Acids (Macronutrients). Institute of Medicine of the National Academies, 2004. http://www.nap.edu/books/0309085373/html/

16. Physical activity, and health: a report of the surgeon general. In: National Center for Chronic Disease Prevention and Health Promotion. Atlanta, GA: US Department of Health and Human Services, Centers for Disease Control and Prevention, 1996, p. 1–4.

17. Pollock ML, Franklin BA, Balady GJ, Chaitman BL, Fleg JL, Fletcher B, Limacher M, Pina IL, Stein RA, Williams M, and Bazzarre T. AHA Science Advisory. Resistance exercise in individuals with and without cardiovascular disease: benefits, rationale, safety, and prescription: an advisory from the Committee on Exercise, Rehabilitation, and Prevention, Council on Clinical Cardiology, American Heart Association; Position paper endorsed by the American College of Sports Medicine. Circulation 101: 828–833, 2000.

18. Miller WC. How effective are traditional dietary and exercise interventions for weight loss? Med Sci Sports Exerc 31: 1129–1134, 1999.

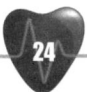

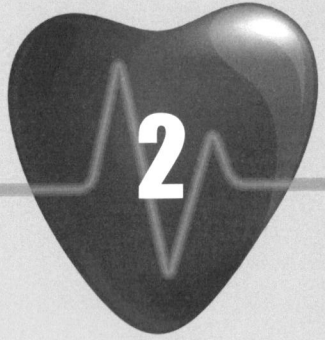

2

WHY EXERCISE?

Aerobic Exercise for Optimum Health

Aerobic Exercise for Optimum Health

Aerobic means "with oxygen" and aerobic exercise refers to exercise which is performed with moderate intensity and is undertaken for at least 20 minutes at an intensity of 70-80% of maximum heart rate. Examples of training aerobically are jogging, swimming, cycling (non-sprint) and the many home (DVD and Broadcast) and fitness studio workouts (usually to music) that have been designed to elevate the heart rate for 20 minutes plus.

The two major goals of aerobic training should be:

1. To develop the capacity of the central circulation system to deliver oxygen to cells.

2. To enhance the capacity of the active musculature to supply and process oxygen.

Why Exercise?

Aerobic Training Health & Lifestyle Benefits

Cardiovascular Adaptations

Aerobic exercise training, because of the intimate link between the cardiovascular system and the aerobic energy process, can dramatically improve cardiovascular function. This is because aerobic training causes increased oxygen delivery to active muscles.

Cardiac Adaptation

Regardless of a person's age, the mass and volume of the heart increases with aerobic training; it becomes stronger and more efficient. This adaptation is the normal muscular response to an increased workload. **However, when aerobic training ceases for a long period of time, the heart loses its thickened, stronger walls and becomes less efficient. The heart is weakened**. [1]

Scientists have compared endurance-trained and resistance-trained athletes to untrained individuals in numerous studies to compare structural and dimensional characteristics of heart changes. **To date, there has been no scientific evidence that indicates that exercise training**

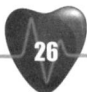

can damage a normal, healthy heart. In fact, based on the results of almost all the research, exercise causes the heart to enlarge and become stronger. The adaptations to regular exercise generally reflected specific training demands. [2, 3]

A heart that becomes larger, with thicker walls, has a superior functional capacity. Exercise 'stress' is only temporary. Exercise provides 'temporary myocardial stress' which can then be stopped by adequate rest times for repair, recuperation and recovery.

Cardiac hypertrophy (excessive development or increase in bulk) is not caused by exercises. It occurs in response to chronic degenerative diseases such as cardiovascular disease or hypertension. These conditions result from the heart having to chronically work against excessive resistance to blood flow. In fact, people who have these debilitating heart conditions that cause hypertrophy are encouraged to exercise to promote heart health. [4, 5, 6]

Plasma Volume Adaptation

A significant change takes place in plasma volume within 24 hours of aerobic exercise. **On average, blood volume increases 12 to 20% after three to six weeks of aerobic exercise**. [7, 8] **Increased blood flow means a better supply of nutrients to all of the organs**.

Heart Rate Adaptation

Aerobic exercise training creates an imbalance or a temporary increase in the sympathetic nervous system activity. Once the exercise ends, the sympathetic system's response is followed by a rise in parasympathetic (PS) activity. [9, 10] This response in the autonomic nervous system (PS activity) following **aerobic training can help to significantly decrease stress levels**.

Stroke Volume Adaptation

Aerobic training causes the heart's stroke volume to increase during rest and exercise. This adaptation response results from a plasma volume increase, improved cardiac muscle usage (reduced stiffness), increased diastolic filling time (the heart becomes more efficient) and improved cardiac contractile function. [11, 12, 13]

What is important to note from scientific studies on aerobic training:

• The hearts of individuals who have endurance-trained exhibit considerably larger stroke volumes than those of untrained individuals.

• The greatest increases in stroke volume adaptation responses to aerobic exercise training occurred during moderate levels of exercise.

Cardiac Output Adaptation

An increase in cardiac output represents the most significant adaptation in cardiovascular function with aerobic training. [14]

Oxygen Extraction Adaptation

Aerobic training significantly increases the quantity of oxygen extracted from circulating blood. [15] This is because the more effective the heart is, the more oxygen is taken into the body (blood oxygenation). **Trained muscle fibres develop an enhanced capacity to extract and process available oxygen**. [16, 17]

The body needs oxygen. Cells quickly become weak and atrophy without regular aerobic training.

Skeletal Muscle Blood Flow Adaptation

Aerobic training increases total skeletal muscle blood flow during exercise. It also enlarges small and large arteries and veins, and causes (on average) a 10% increase in capillarisation per gram of muscle tissue. [18, 19]

Myocardial Blood Flow Adaptation

Aerobic training adaptation responses to myocardial blood flow include an increase in the cross-sectional area of proximal coronary arteries and an increase in capillary density. These adaptation responses alone can dramatically support the necessary blood flow and energy demands of possibly the most important organ in the body, the heart. [20, 21, 22, 23]

Sustained, aerobic, endurance training specifically increases coronary blood flow and improves myocardial vascularisation when new capillaries form and develop into small arterioles. [24, 25]

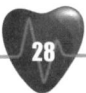

Blood Pressure

Regular aerobic training reduces systolic and diastolic blood pressures during rest and exercise training. The largest decrease usually occurs in systolic pressure in individuals with high blood pressure.

A brisk walking programme may not provide a satisfactory stimulus to evoke a positive adaptation response. [26, 27, 28, 29, 30, 31, 32] Regular aerobic training however, can help to control the tendency for blood pressure to rise in those at risk from hypertension (high blood pressure). It can also promote adequate stimulus for positive heart changes. [33]

Pulmonary Adaptations

Aerobic training stimulates adaptations in pulmonary (lung) ventilation. This may be due to a particular breathing strategy during exercise, which minimises respiratory work. However, research suggests that oxygen is made available for use by the non-respiratory active muscular system. [34, 35]

Scientific studies of people of all ages have consistently shown positive training adaptations in pulmonary ventilation from moderate aerobic exercise training. [36, 37]

Metabolic Adaptations

Endurance-trained skeletal muscle contains more and larger mitochondria than less active muscle fibre. The increased and enlarged number of mitochondria means adenosine triphosphate (ATP) production becomes more efficient and this means **higher energy and better health**. [38, 39]

Fat Metabolism

Aerobic endurance training increases the capability to burn fat as it increases the individual's capacity to mobilise and deliver (oxidise) fatty acids for energy consumption during exercise. [40, 41, 42]

Endurance-trained muscle also benefits from further metabolic adaptations:

• Greater blood flow within trained muscles.

• More fat-metabolising enzymes.

• Enhanced muscle mitochondrial respiratory capability.

Aerobic training improves fatty acid oxidation and respiratory ATP production, which improves cell function.

Other Aerobic Adaptation Responses

For overweight or obese individuals, regular aerobic training can reduce body mass and body fat. For best results, combine exercise with healthy nutritional habits. **Endurance-trained individuals can experience profound psychological benefits including improved mood, self-esteem and self-concept and a heightened ability to manage stress**.

In Summary:

•   **Aerobic exercise is a key component of a healthy lifestyle.**

•   **If you fail to undertake regular aerobic exercise your heart will become progressively weaker, laying you open to chronic or life-threatening disease.**

•   **Regular aerobic activity can lower your blood pressure, improve the health of your heart and greatly reduce your stress levels.**

•   **Combined with a healthy diet, aerobic training is an important factor in reducing body fat and thereafter maintaining a healthy body.**

Chapter References

1. Hickson RC, et al. Reduced training intensities and loss of aerobic power, endurance, and cardiac growth. J Appl Physiol 1985;58:492.

2. Effron MB. Effects of resistive training on left ventricular function. Med Sci Sports Exerc 1989;21:694.

3. Plumm BM, et al. The athlete's heart: a meta-analysis of cardiac structure. Circulation 2000;101:336.

4. Bennet DH, et a l. Echocardiographic left ventricular dimensions in pressure and volume overload. Their use in assessing aortic stenosis. Br heart J 1975;37:971.

5. Mitchell JH, et al. How to recognize "athletes heart." Phys. Sportsmed 1992;20(8):87.

6. Sawka MN, et al. Blood volume: importance and adaptations to exercise training, environmental stresses, and trauma/sickness. Med Sci Sports Exerc

2000;32:332.

7. Hagberg. JM. Expanded blood volumes contribute to increased cardiovascular performance of endurance-trained older men. J Appl Physiol 1998;85:484.

8. Goldsmith RL, et al. Physical fitness as a determinant of vagal modulation. Med Sci Sports Exerc 1997;29:812.

9. Shin K, et al. Autonomic differences between athletes and non athletes: spectral analysis approach. Med Sci Sports Exerc 1997;29:1482.

10. Krip B, et al. Effect of alterations in blood volume on cardiac function during maximal exercise. Med Sci Sports Exerc 1997;29:1496.

11. Mier CM, et al. Cardiovascular adaptations to 10 days of cycle exercise. J Appl Physiol 1997;83:1900.

12. Loftin M, et al. Effects of arm training on central and peripheral circulatory function. Med Sci Sports Exerc 1988;20:136.

13. Cunningham DA, et al. Development of cardiorespiratory function in circumpubertal boys: a longitudinal study. J Appl Physiol 1984;56:302.

14. Rowell LB. Human cardiovascular control. Cary, NC: Oxford University Press, 1994.

15. Lakatta EG. Cardiovascular regulatory mechanisms in advanced age. Physiol Rev 1993;73:413.

16. Seals DR, et al. Exercise and aging: autonomic control of the circulation. Med Sci Sports Exerc 1994; 26:568.

17. Hepple RT. Skeletal muscle: microcirculatory adaptation to metabolic demand. Med Sci Sports Exerc 2000;32;117.

18. Lash JM, et al. Exercise training effects on collateral and microvascular resistance in rat model of arterial insufficiency. Am J Physiol 1995;28:H125.

19. Hambrecht R, et al. Effect of exercise on coronary endothelial function in patients with coronary artery disease. N. Engl J Med 2000;342:454.

20. Laughlin MH, et al. Control of blood flow to cardiac and skeletal muscle during exercise, In: Rowell LB, Shepherd JT, eds. Handbook of physiology, exercise: regulation and integration of multiple systems. Bethesda, MD: American Physiological Society, 1996.

21. Moore RL, Palmer BM. Exercise training and cellular adaptations of normal and diseased hearts. Exerc Sport Sci Rev 1999;27:285.

22. White FC, et al. Exercise training in swine promotes growth of arteriolar bed and capillary angiogenesis in heart. J Appl Physiol 1998;85:1160.

23. Laughlin MH, et al. McAllister RM. Exercise training-induced coronary vascular adaptation. J Appl Physiol 1992;73:2209.

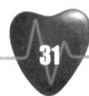

24. Baglivo HP, et al. Effect of moderate physical training on left ventricular mass in mild hypertensive persons. Hypertension 1990;15(Suppl.I):1.

25. Dengel DR, et al. Improvements in blood pressure, glucose metabolism, and lipoprotein lipids after aerobic exercise plus weight loss in obese, hypertensive middle-aged men. Metabolism 1998;47:1075.

26. Hagberg JM. Physical activity, physical fitness, and blood pressure. In: Leon A, ed. Physical activity and cardiovascular health. Champaign, IL: Human Kinetics, 1997.

27. Kraemer WJ, et al. Resistance training combined with bench-step aerobics enhances women's health profile. Med Sci Sports Exerc 2001;33:259.

28. O'Conner PJ, et al. State anxiety and ambulatory blood pressure following resistance training exercises in females. Med Sci Sports Exerc 1993;25:516.

29. Urata H et al. Antihypertensive and volume-depleting effects of mild exercise on essential hypertension. Hypertension 1987;9:245.

30. Wilmore JH, et al. Heart rate and blood pressure changes with endurance training: The Heritage Family Study. Med Sci Sports Exerc 2001;33:107.

31. Paffenbarger RS Jr, et al. Physical activity and hypertension: an epidemiological view. Ann Med 1991;23:19.

32. McConnell AK, Semple, ESG. Ventilatory sensitivity to carbon dioxide: the influence of exercise and athleticism. Med Sci Sports Exerc 1996;28:685, 1996.

33. Taylor R, Jones N. The reduction by training of CO2 output during exercise. Eur J Cardiol 1979;9:53.

34. Jirka Z, Adamus M. Changes of ventilation equivalents in young people in the course of three years of training. J Sports Med 1965;5:1.

35. Tzankoff SP, et al. Physiological adjustments to work in older men as affected by physical training. J Appl Physiol 1972;33:346.

36. Hickson RC. Skeletal muscle cytochrome c and myoglobin, endurance, and frequency of training. J Appl Physiol 1981;51:746.

37. Holloszy JO. Metabolic consequences of endurance exercise training. In: Horton ES, Terjung RL, eds. Exercise, nutrition, and energy metabolism. New York: Macmillan, 1988.

38. Coggan AR, et al. Isotopic estimation of CO2 production during exercise before and after endurance training. J Appl Physiol 1993;75:70.

39. Friedlander AL, et al. Training-induced alterations of carbohydrate metabolism in women; women respond differently than men. J Appl Physiol 1998;85:1175.

40. Horowitz JF. Regulation of lipid mobilization and oxidation during exercise in obesity. Exer Sport Sci Revs 2001;29:42

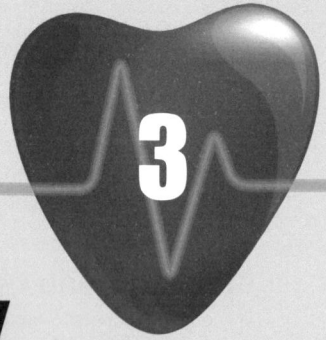

WHY
EXERCISE?

3

**Anaerobic Training for
Optimum Health**

Anaerobic Training for Optimum Health

Because anaerobic training is more stressful on the body than aerobic training, the adaptation responses to the physiology of the heart (health benefits) are different. This is why both anaerobic and aerobic training are necessary.

Scientific research has shown anaerobic training causes the central wall of the heart (the septum) to become thicker. **This adaptation response can lower the risk of cardiovascular disease**. However, it is important to note here that too much anaerobic training (or overtraining in general) can be very harmful on the body, as it loses its acid-alkaline balance and becomes more acidic. High pH levels are very dangerous and can result in serious illnesses.

Anaerobic training places a stress on the cardiorespiratory system. Regardless of the duration and/or intensity, we use the cardiorespiratory system to sustain the activity for short periods of time. We also need the cardiorespiratory system to recuperate from training. [1, 2, 3, 4]

Cardiorespiratory exercise can have a profound effect on the overall physical and mental health of an individual. [5, 6, 7-15] It can decrease the risk of developing hypertension, cancer, osteoporosis, obesity, non-insulin dependant diabetes, coronary artery disease (CAD), anxiety levels and daily fatigue.

Overload of the anaerobic system stimulates metabolic adaptations in anaerobic function. This primarily brings about changes in the immediate and short-term energy systems.

We derive energy from anaerobic and aerobic energy metabolic pathways. However, our ability to use these pathways varies from person to person. Furthermore, energy transfer capabilities are not related to general fitness levels, but depend on the specific type of exercise in which the individual is involved. [16, 17, 18, 19]

How we Produce Fuel for Exercise

There are three main bio-energetic pathways that produce the fuel for our bodies – adenosine triphosphate (ATP). [20-25] Some exercise physiologists and scientists refer to this as the bio-energetic continuum.

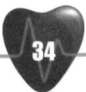

The Three Pathways

• ATP-CP (Creatine Phosphate) – An anaerobic pathway, used with high intensity, short duration exercise (for example, an all-out 100 metre sprint).

• Glycolysis (Lactate Acid) – An anaerobic pathway, used with a moderate to high intensity activity (for example, a 200 metre sprint).

• Oxidative (Oxygen) – An aerobic pathway, used with a low to moderate intensity activity (for example, jogging for 20 - 30 minutes).

Different durations and intensities of effort activate the appropriate energy pathways. However, it is difficult to place any activity in a specific energy pathway. As an individual develops greater levels of anaerobic fitness, what once was anaerobic for them may become aerobic.

The ATP-CP and Glycolysis energy systems largely power any exercise up to 2 minutes. These systems require oxygen. A need for anaerobic energy exists for fast and short-duration movements. [26]

Use It or Lose It

When an individual stops exercising regularly, a loss in physiological and performance adaptations rapidly occurs. [27]

Anaerobic Training

Speed and agility training can be strenuous. To avoid injuries while training anaerobically, individuals should build up speed gradually, and never abruptly. This will help to avoid risk of injury to bones, joints and muscles. [28, 29]

Intensity

Intensity depends on many factors including age, gender, skill, bodyweight and motivation. It requires the individual to be focused. Students can also learn to use the rating of perceived exertion (RPE). [30, 31] This psychophysiologic approach was first developed by Gunnar Borg, and encourages students to "listen to their own body".

Children

Do not push children too hard anaerobically. It is unclear why anaerobic capabilities are lower in children. One possible reason involves their

slower rate of glycogen use during exercise. [32, 33] Whatever the reason, adapt your training to the lower-capacity for anaerobic training in children.

In Summary:

- **Anaerobic training is just as important as aerobic training for your overall health, especially for your heart, however, in moderation.**

- **Correct anaerobic training for your level of physical ability is a vital component in the fight against many chronic or life threatening conditions.**

- **However, watch out for the telltale signs that you may be pushing yourself too hard (overtraining). If you should feel sluggish or lacking in motivation, try scaling back your anaerobic training until you regain your previous energy levels.**

- **Always ensure that you warm up thoroughly before training anaerobically and that you avoid jerky movements that may overstretch your joint and ligaments. Build up speed and power progressively and, above all, listen to what your body is telling you.**

Chapter References

1. Holly RG, Shaffrath JD. Cardiorespiratory endurance. Chapter 52. In American College of Sports Medicine (ed.).

ACSM's resource manual for guidelines for exercise testing and prescription. 3rd edition. Baltimore, MD: Williams & Wilkins; 1998.

2. Brooks GA, Fahey TD, White TP. Exercise physiology: human bioenergetics and its application. 2nd edition.

Moutain View, CA: Mayfield Publishing Company; 1996.

3. Greenhaff PL, Timmons JA. Interaction between aerobic and anaerobic metabolism during intense muscle contraction. In Holsey JO, (ed).

4. Exercise and Sport Science Reviews. Volume . Baltimore: Williams & Wilkins;1998. pp. 1-30.

5. Holly RG, Shaffrath JD. Cardiorespiratory endurance. Chapter 52. In American College of Sports Medicine (ed.). ACSM's resource manual for guidelines for exercise testing and prescription. 3rd edition. Baltimore, MD:

Williams & Wilkins; 1998.

6. Brooks GA, Fahey TD, White TP. Exercise physiology: human bioenergetics and its application. 2nd edition. Moutain View, CA: Mayfield Publishing Company; 1996.

7. Pate RR, Pratt MM, Blair SN, Haskell WL, Macera CA, Bouchard C, Buchner D, Ettinger W, Heath GW, King AC. Physical activity and public health: a recommendation from the Centers for Disease Control and Prevention and the American College of Sports Medicine. JAMA 1995; 273:402-7.

8. Lambert EV, Bohlmann I, Cowling K. Physical activity for health: understanding the epidemiological evidence for risk benefits. Int Sport Med J 2001;1(5):1-15.

9. Blair SN, Wei M. Sedentary habits, health, and function in older women and men. Am J Health Promot 2000;15(1):1-8.

10. Blair SN, Kohl HW, Barlow CE, Paffenbarger RS Jr, Gibbons LW, Macera CA. Changes in physical fitness and all-cause mortality. A prospective study of healthy and unhealthy men. JAMA 1995;273(14):1093-8.

11. Blair SN. Physical inactivity and cardiovascular disease risk in women. Med Sci Sports Exerc 1996;28(1):9-10.

12. Smolander J, Blair SN, Kohl HW 3rd. Work ability, physical activity, and cardiorespiratory fitness: 2-year results from Project Active. J Occup Environ Med 2000;42(9):906-10.

13. American College of Sports Medicine. ACSM's guidelines for exercise testing and prescription. 5th edition. Philadelphia: Williams & Wilkins; 1995.

14. Wei M, Schwertner HA, Blair SN. The association between physical activity, physical fitness, and type 2 diabetes mellitus. Compr Ther 2000;26(3):176-82.

15. Andreoli A, Monteleone M, Van Loan M, Promenzio L, Tarantino U, De Lorenzo A. Effects of different sports on bone density and muscle mass in highly trained athletes. Med Sci Sports Exerc 2001;33(4):507-11.

16. Magel. JR, et al. Specificity of swim training on maximum oxygen uptake. J Appl Physiol 1975;38:151.

17. Magel JR, et al. Metabolic and cardiovascular adjustment to arm training. J Appl Physiol 1978;45:75.

18. McArdle WD, et al. Comparison of continuous and discontinuous treadmill and bicycle tests for max VO2 Med Sci Sport 1973;5:156.

19. Pechar GS, et al. Specificity of cardiorespiratory adaptation to bicycle and treadmill training. J Appl Physiol 1974;36:753.

20. Brooks GA, Fahey TD, White TP. Exercise physiology: human bioenergetics and its application. 2nd edition. Moutain View, CA: Mayfield Publishing Company; 1996.

21. Hicks GH. Cardiopulmonary anatomy and physiology. Philadelphia: W.B. Saunders Company; 2000.

22. American College of Sports Medicine. ACSM's guidelines for exercise testing and prescription. 5th edition. Philadelphia: Williams & Wilkins; 1995.

23. Greenhaff PL, Timmons JA. Interaction between aerobic and anaerobic metabolism during intense muscle contraction. In Holsey JO, (ed). Exercise and Sport Science Reviews. Volume 26. Baltimore: Williams & Wilkins; 1998. pp. 1 to 30.

24. Stone MH, Conley MS. Bioenergetics. Chapter 5. In Baechle TR (ed.). Essentials of strength training and conditioning. Champaign, IL: Human Kinetics; 1994.

25. Volek JS. Enhancing exercise performance: nutritional implications. Chapter 32. In Garrett WE, Kirkendall DT (eds.). Exercise and sport science. Philadelphia: Lippincott Williams & Wilkins; 2000.

26. Koziris LB, et al. Relationship of aerobic power to anaerobic performance indices. J strength Cond Res 1996;10:35.

27. Mukija I, Padilla S. Cardiorespiratory and metabolic characteristics of detraining in humans. Med Sci Sports Exerc 2001;33:413.

28. Almeida SA, et al. Epidemiological patterns of musculoskeletal injuries and physical training. Med. Sci Sports Exerc 1999;31:1176.

29. Jones BH, et al. Epidemiology of injuries associated with physical training among young men in the army. Med Sci Sports Exerc 1993;25:197.

30. Borg GA. Psychological basis of physical exertion. Med Sci Sports Exerc 1982;14:377.

31. Robertson RJ, Noble BJ. Perception of physical exertion: methods, mediators, and applications. Exerc Sport Sci. Rev 1997;25:407.

32. Bowles DK, et al. Coronary smooth muscle and endothelial adaptations to exercise training. Exerc Sport Sci Rev 2000;28:57.

33. Delp MD, Laughlin MH. Time course of enhanced endothelium-mediated dilation in aorta of trained rats. Med Sci Sports Exerc 1997;29:1454.

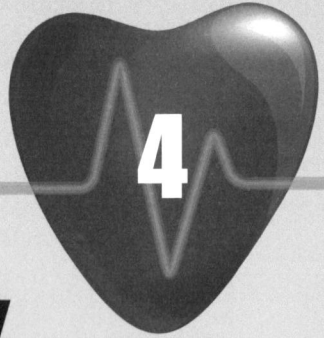

WHY
EXERCISE?

Resistance Training for Optimum Health

Resistance Training for Optimum Health

Resistance training can improve balance, speed, endurance and power. It can also help an individual to become mentally stronger, healthier overall, and less prone to injury. Resistance training involves bodyweight, free weights or weight training machine exercises.

Goals for Resistance Training

Resistance training exercises can improve the body's condition and help the person to recover faster between workouts. A strong body is better able to fight off illnesses and disease. Also, a person who is strong physically, usually feels more confident mentally.

When implementing resistance training exercises (RTE) into an exercise programme it is important to train the whole body, weekly. Your exercise programme should aim to strengthen the entire body, all joints, muscles, tendons and ligaments, weekly. Greater strength can improve levels of endurance and stamina too.

A Brief History of Resistance Training

Resistance training has had a slow acceptance in the fitness world. The concept first became well known in the 1950s. At this time, many competitive weight lifters, body-builders and athletes started training using resistance or weight-lifting exercises. However, at that time, many athletes believed that resistance training which added muscle would slow them down. They also thought that added muscle would cause a loss in joint flexibility and would somehow "turn to fat" once their competitive careers were over.

Such myths perpetuated until the 1960s. Finally, documented research clearly illustrated the truth about resistance training. Today, countless scientific studies have proven the benefits of resistance training. It improves strength, speed, power, endurance and joint flexibility.

Some Truths about Resistance Training

As we mentioned, there have been many misconceptions about resistance training. But let's look at some of the facts that science has proven about this type of exercise.

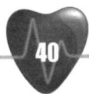

Strength and Gender

Generally, men possess considerably greater strength than women in all muscle groups. Women usually score 50% lower than men in upper-body strength tests and about 30% less for leg strength. [1] Of course, there are exceptions. For instance, professional female track-and-field athletes who have trained for years are usually stronger than untrained men.

Training Muscles to Become Stronger & Healthier

When a muscle is forced to work harder with each resistance-based repetition, it is progressively "overloaded". In order to exert enough strength to finish the exercise, the muscle is forced to gain strength.

Overload intensity is the level of tension put on the muscle. Any exercise that puts enough tension on the muscle to cause overload will improve strength. As mentioned for health, your aim should be to use RTEs to strengthen the entire body for wellness and longevity.

Understanding Resistance Training

A concentric action occurs as a muscle shortens. For example, when performing a biceps curl, lifting the weight upward shortens the biceps.

An eccentric action occurs as a muscle lengthens. For example, lowering the weights in a biceps curl. This eccentric action also helps to lengthen and stretch the muscle.

Combined concentric and eccentric muscle actions are the essence of resistance training. Through these two activities, muscular strength is improved. [2, 3] However, eccentric muscle contractions are more likely to cause soreness and injury. However, data suggests that eccentric overload training is more effective at preserving strength gains. [4]

Types of Resistance Training

Weight Lifting

The most popular form of resistance training is probably weight-lifting, usually with free weights or machines at a health/fitness club. This method selectively strengthens specific muscles by causing them to

overcome resistance.

Bodyweight Exercises
Bodyweight exercises are excellent for developing whole body strength, because they simultaneously improve balance and core strength.

Progressive Resistance Exercises
When incorporating resistance exercises into any fitness programme, remember to build your strength gradually. This technique is called progressive resistance exercises (PRE). In particular, avoid maximum repetitions, (performing to muscular failure) because excessive resistance training greatly increases the risk of muscle and joint injury. Remember to gradually strengthen muscles, joints, tendons and ligaments with progressive increases while resistance training.

Competitive athletes often focus on maximising strength gains when performing resistance training exercises. But **scientific studies have concluded that adults who focused on 'maintaining' their overall health and physical fitness improved their muscular strength, endurance and bone mass by light, progressive resistance training**. [5, 6, 7, 8, 9]

Let's take a closer look at the goal of "optimal health". Resistance training by itself plays only a small part in improving cardiovascular fitness. It's not enough to avoid heart disease risk factors. [10] On the positive side, intense resistance training can cause a small blood volume increase (during exercises, more oxygen can travel to the muscles for fuel and to the skin for cooling). [11] However, for long-term health purposes, scientific data shows that the major portion of a workout should not be resistance-based. Evidence suggests that less than 10% of the total workout time should be spent on resistance training.

How Strength Gains Occur
Scientists do not fully understand how strength is built. However, there are several important factors to building strength and stamina. Let's look at the factors that are understood.

The Nervous System's Role
Although many studies have been done to explain the effects of resistance training on the development of muscle, there are holes in

the knowledge. Basically, scientists have noted that the early stages of resistance exercise training show extremely fast muscle strength gains. This rapid response can't be caused by only muscle-based mechanisms. In fact, research suggests that the nervous system is involved.

Resistance training specifically develops strength from the way the nerves are organised between the brain and the muscles. When the motor units are excited by activity, the muscle fibre itself quickly adapts. [12, 13, 14]

A muscle's ability to generate force depends on factors related to the nervous system. When a person's brain sends a "move" signal to a particular group of muscles, the nervous system transmits this message then recruits and fires the correct motor units. However, when the muscles respond, the amount of force they can generate also depends on the muscle fibre types. [15, 16, 17, 18]

A person can improve this communication between the brain and muscles. By repeatedly practicing movements, the body fine-tunes that signal and response time. The improvement means more speed, power and strength.

This results in:

- Greater neuromuscular efficiency
- Improved motor unit synchronisation
- Increased CNS activation
- **Greater circulation and overall health**

Environmental Factors

Scientific studies show that many environmental factors affect human muscular strength. Stress prevents people from expressing their true strength capability. [19]

The Relationship between Strength, Power and Speed

There is an inherent relationship between a muscle's ability to produce power and the rate at which it contracts (or contraction speed). Strength increases improve power increases; and as power improves, so does speed.

During resistance exercise training, muscular tension increases are

the main reason muscles grow (hypertrophy). The mechanical stress, or overloading, stimulates increases in muscle size. [20, 21] However, as mentioned earlier, neurological factors affect human strength. So, strength and power increases do not necessarily require muscles to grow. Therefore, people with certain muscle fibre types that don't easily "bulk up" can still see a great increase in power, strength and overall health.

Connective Tissue Improvements

Resistance training has a side-benefit of thickening and strengthening connective tissue. Ligaments and tendons become structurally and functionally more efficient. [22] These changes protect muscles and joints from injury, and this research justifies the use of resistance training exercises for rehabilitation programmes, and for optimum health purposes.

Age Factors

Age does not affect the muscles' responses to the stimulus of training. In scientific studies, older men and women adapted to both resistance and endurance training. [23] Women and men can also benefit from the psychological responses to resistance training. [23, 24, 25, 26]

Muscle Soreness

During and after exercise, the degree of muscle soreness a person experiences depends on the fitness of the individual, the intensity and duration of the exercise and the type of exercise performed. [27, 28, 10] Muscle soreness usually results from active strains on muscle fibres during heavy-resistance overload training. [11]

Strength Maintenance

In scientific studies, one or two weekly resistance-based workout sessions proved to be enough stimuli for maintaining training-induced strength and health gains. [28]

Core Strength

The deep transverse abdominal muscles that wrap around the abdomen (and also connect to the rib cage) stabilise the core and work to maintain the correct alignment of the spine. Prolonged lack of use often results in

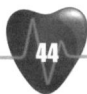

poor function and control of this important muscle group, which can lead to a variety of musculoskeletal problems. The muscles of the core are composed of a high proportion of slow twitch muscle fibres, which have good endurance capabilities. RTEs that strengthen the deep abdominal muscles of the core are essential in any exercise programme.

Physiological Adaptations to Resistance Training [29]

Muscle Fibres

Size – Increase

Strength – Increase

Connective Tissue

Ligament Strength – Increase

Tendon Strength – Increase

Bone Mineral Content and Density - Increase

Mitochondria

Volume – Decrease

Density – Decrease

Capillary Density

No change, or some slight decrease

Modified from Komi PV, ed. Strength and power in sport. London: Blackwell Scientific, 1992.

Because the decrease in mitochondria and capillary density associated with resistance training is not favourable, resistance training should only be a part of a complete, holistic exercise programme. Too much resistance or strength training can be harmful.

Resistance Training with Children

Little research has been conducted concerning the benefits and risks of resistance training with children. However, some carefully conducted research showed that resistance training with high repetitions and low resistance significantly improved muscular strength in children.

In Summary:

- **Resistance training is an important element for you in creating a stronger, disease-resistant body, improved endurance and stamina and a more confident mental attitude as well.**

- **Don't be mislead by outdated myths. Correct resistance training does NOT slow you down or make you stiff and inflexible – and muscle does NOT "turn to fat" if you should stop exercising!**

- **It's never too soon, or too late, to start with proper guidance. Progressive resistance training will help you to strengthen your body and delay or even avoid many common health problems, whatever your age.**

Chapter References

1. Heyward VH, et al. Gender differences in strength. Res Q Exerc Sport 1986;57:154.

2. Hather BM, et al. Influence of eccentric actions on skeletal muscle adaptations to resistance training. Acta Physiol Scand 1991;143:177.

3. O'Hagan FT, et al. Comparative effectiveness of accommodating and weight resistance training modes. Med Sci Sports Exerc 1995;27:1210.

4. Colliander EB, Tesch, PA, Effects of detraining following short term resistance training on eccentric and concentric muscle strength. Acta Physiol Scand. 1992;144:23.

5. Exercise training guidelines for the elderly. Med Sci Sports Exerc 1999;31:12.

6. Hurley BF, Hagberg JM. Optimizing health in older persons; aerobic or strength training? Exerc Sport Sci Rev 1998;26:61.

7. Layne JE, Nelson ME. The effects of progressive resistance training on bone density: a review. Med Sci Sports Exerc 1999;31:25.

8. Lemmer JT, et al. Effect of strength training on resting metabolic rate and physical activity: age and gender comparisons. Med Sci Sports Exerc 2001;33:532.

9. Wescott WL, Baechle TR. Strength training past 50. Champaign, IL: Human Kinetics, 1998.

10. Pizza FX, et al. Exercise-induced muscle damage: effect on circulating leukocyte and lymphocyte subset. Med Sci Sports Exerc 1995;27:363.

11. Lieber RL. Friden J. Muscle damage is not a function of muscle force but active muscle strain. J Appl Physiol 1993;74:520.

12. Narici M, et al. Human quadriceps cross-sectional area, torque, and neural activation during 6 months speed training. Acta Physiol Scand 1996;1547:175.

13. Prevost MC, et al. The effect of two days of velocity-specific isokinetic training on torque production. J Strength Cond Res 1999;13:35.

14. Staron RS, et al. Skeletal muscle adaptations during the early phase of heavy-resistance training in men and women. J Appl Pysiol 1994;76:1247.

15. Conley MS, et al. Resistance training and human cervical muscle recruitment plasticity. J Appl Physiol 1997;83:2105.

16. Kellis E, Blatzopoulos V. Muscle activation differences between eccentric and concentric isokinetic exercise. Med Sci Sports Exerc 1998;30:1616.

17. O' Hagan FT, et al. Comparative effectiveness of accommodating and weight resistance training modes. Med Sci Sports Exerc 1995;27:1210.

18. Sleivert GG, et al. The influence of strength-sprint training sequence on multi-joint power output. Med Sci Sports Exerc 1995;27:1655.

19. Ikai M, Steinhaus AH. Some factors modifying the expression of human strength. J Appl Physiol 1961;16:157.

20. Carson JA. The regulation of gene expression in hypertrophying skeletal muscle. Exerc Sport Sci Rev 1997;25:301.

21. Charette SL, et al. Muscle hypertrophy response to resistance training in older women. J Appl Physiol 1991;70:912.

22. Vailas AC, Vailas JC. Physical activity and connective tissue. In: Bouchard C, et al., eds. Physical activity, fitness and health. Champaign, IL: Human Kinetics, 1994.

23. Coggan AR, et al. Skeletal muscle adaptations to endurance training in 60 to 70 year old men and women. J Appl Physiol 1992;72:1780.

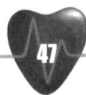

24. Roman WJ, et al. Adaptations in the elbow flexors of elderly males after resistance training. J Appl Physiol 1993;74:750.

25. Sipala S. Suominen H. Effects of strength and endurance training on thigh and leg muscle mass and composition in elderly women. J Appl Physiol 1995;78:334.

26. Yarasheski KE, et al. Acute effects of resistance exercise on muscle protein synthesis in young and eldery adults. Am J Physiol 1993;265:E210.

27. Duarte JA, et al. Exercise-induced signs of muscle overuse in children. Int J Sports Med 1999;20:103.

28. Graves JE, e al. Effect of reduced training frequency on muscular strength. Int J Sports Med 1988;9:316.

29. Modified from Fleck SJ, Kramer WJ. Resistance training: physiological responses and adaptations (part 2 of 4). Phys Sportsmed, 1988;16:108.

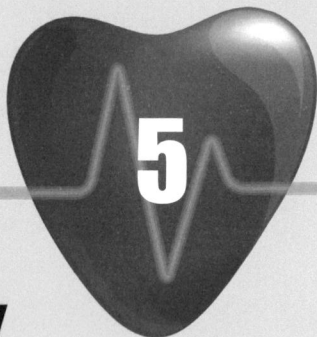

WHY
EXERCISE?

Stretching/Flexibility Training for Optimum Health

Stretching/Flexibility Training for Optimum Health

The ability to move your muscles and joints through their full range of motion (ROM) is flexibility.

How can a person achieve greater-than average flexibility levels and increased ROM in joints? By performing a whole-body, yoga-based stretch.

Every person can become more limber by stretching regularly using a whole-body stretch. However, very often people have limited flexibility in specific areas of the body. For example, they might have tight hamstrings and poor leg flexibility, but great shoulder flexibility.

Flexibility can be gained and lost and sedentary lifestyles cramp our muscles. Individuals who spend large amounts of time sitting in front of computers or televisions usually have tight, uncooperative muscles and stiffness in the neck, back and shoulder joints. This is because inactivity causes a steady loss of flexibility, so people should be discouraged from stretching for a few months and then stopping. **Many doctors and scientists are now stating that regular stretching for a lifetime is compulsory for optimum health.**

The Lifestyle Factor
Obviously, an active person will be more flexible than an individual who is less active. Poor lifestyle habits have a negative effect on an individual's flexibility.

Overall Flexibility
Greater levels of overall flexibility can contribute to an improved feeling of well-being and, therefore, better enjoyment in every area of life.

Understanding Stretching/Flexibility Training
Your skeletal muscles move your body by contracting and relaxing, thus pulling on bones to create movement. If muscles and surrounding tissues are flexible and elastic, the joint can move through its full range-of-motion (ROM). The opposite is true if muscles and surrounding tissues are inflexible and tight.

Bones, Joints and Connective Tissue

Flexibility is not just dependent on how elastic muscle tissue is; ligaments and tendons contribute significantly. Muscles, body fat levels and even skin all play a part in flexibility.

The Nervous System

The autonomic nervous system's main function is to make sure the body stays in balance. This is called homeostasis, and it helps ensure that basic needs – such as hunger and thirst – are met. This balance regulates the body activities without conscious control.

The autonomic nervous system is divided into two categories: the sympathetic nervous system (SNS) and the parasympathetic nervous system (PSNS). The SNS and PSNS are primarily distinguished by their opposite effects on the body's organs and systems.

Aerobic and anaerobic training stimulates the SNS, thus using the stored energy of the body. On the other hand, the PSNS is activated during the absence of stress. When it's activated, one of the things it stimulates is the body's reserves. That is why stretching can create a sense of calmness and peace. Activation of the PSNS helps individuals to relax, allows us to take in minerals and vitamins better, and builds new healthy cells.

When the PSNS is activated through stretching, the body reacts:

• **Heart beat slows down**

• **Blood pressure decreases**

• **Blood vessels dilate**

• **Breathing becomes slower and easier**

• **Stomach secretion increases**

• **Immune system function increases**

Methods of Stretching

Today, there are several popular methods of stretching, with static, yoga-based stretching being the most popular.

Dynamic Stretching

This method of stretching is accomplished by performing a movement, like rising leg swings, through a full range of motion at an increased speed, but <u>not</u> at ballistic speeds. Ballistic stretching, once popular, is risky and injuries are common.

Static Stretching

Static stretching involves lengthening a muscle/muscle group and then holding the stretch for 20-30 seconds or longer. However, with this process, muscles will only lengthen to the degree of the ROM in the accommodating joints.

This method of stretching is easy to perform and very relaxing. It has an extremely low risk of injury and many health benefits.

Performing Stretching Exercises Correctly

Whatever method of stretching you partake in for your health, stretches must be correctly executed to be beneficial. For example, one common mistake with static stretching exercises is to round the spine while leg stretching. Another common error is to bend the knees in order to stretch further. These errors cause the muscles or muscle groups to be actually stretched less. Performing a stretch incorrectly can also damage muscles, or more commonly, joints or connective tissue. Stretching exercises should never be painful. Anyone doing a stretch who feels pain should stop immediately.

In static stretching, try to relax fully. Relaxing into stretches is essential. Some common mistakes -- such as stretching too fast or hard, stretching too suddenly, or bouncing a muscle -- will make muscles contract and tighten.

Management of Stress & Tension

Stress often manifests itself in muscles as tightness. For example, stiff necks and headaches are usually bodily signs of too much stress held in the body.

Tension in the mind often shows quickly in the body. Generally, many people are tense. You can see tension in their face, in their eyes, in how they walk, and even how they speak. **Tension held in the muscles**

reduces circulation, which results in a lack of much needed oxygen. This results in an unfortunate build-up of waste by-products in the muscles. Tense muscles can make flexibility training an ongoing chore and struggle. However, with dedication and time, students can learn to relax tense muscles and better manage their stress.

Reducing Muscle Soreness

Every day, people do many things that can lead to muscle soreness. For example, a shop assistant who goes out to play football with his sons may find himself aching. A typist who paints a bedroom may use muscles in new ways, causing pain. A stretch before and after unusual activities can alleviate some of the discomfort.

In the same way, as we age, our bodies can take longer to recover from training. **Regular stretching can help to reduce muscle soreness by removing waste byproducts from the cells**.

Preventing and Fixing Muscle Imbalances [1, 2, 3, 4]

Every muscle in the body has an optimum length-tension relationship (OL-TR). Muscles need to maintain their OL-TRs to avoid negative impact on joints. When muscles lose their optimum length-tension, muscle imbalances occur. This, consequently, affects the alignment of joints. Sadly today, muscle imbalances are at epidemic levels.

Muscles should create force equally on both sides of the joints they surround. This prevents injury and maintains the way the joint functions. Joint dysfunctions due to muscle imbalances cause excessive stress on joints, ligaments and tendons. This long-term stress causes excessive wear and tear and leads to arthritis, pain, and in many cases, eventual surgery.

Static stretching exercises can work to correct muscle imbalances and to enable joints to become realigned.

Injury Prevention

Obviously, not all injuries are preventable; however, risks can be minimised. When your body is more flexible, it is better able to respond to a sudden slip or fall.

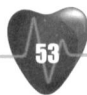

Utilise Deep Abdominal Breathing (DAB) while Stretching

We breathe automatically, many times a minute. But this doesn't mean we breathe efficiently or correctly. Most people only use a small part of their respiratory capacity and lungs, and take shallow, incomplete breaths. While exercising, many people limit their intake of oxygen by closing their mouths and breathing predominantly through their noses.

Dr. Samuel West D.N., founder of The World Wide Blood Protein Research Society, researched the importance of the role of oxygen in our system. He suggests proper oxygenation of the body can help to heal many major illnesses. His scientific research led him to conclude that many diseases stem from the accumulation of cellular debris, toxins and especially excess fluid in the spaces around the body's cells. This build-up prevents the cell from getting enough oxygen to fuel its functions. This occurs especially when there is an inadequate intake of oxygen through the lungs.

Dr. West concluded that DAB activates the lymphatic system (responsible for flushing the body of waste by-products) while the oxygen stimulates the sodium-potassium pump that provides electrical energy for the functioning of the entire body.

The Lymphatic System

The lymphatic system is a major part of the immune system; it helps to provide vital protection from infectious diseases. It also works to prevent the malfunction of internal tissues. This system is compromised of various tissues, vessels and nodes and contains white blood cells. However, it does not have a pump (like the heart in the cardiovascular system). Instead, the lymphatic system is activated and stimulated by proper breathing.

Circulation

Exercise Physiologists have found that flexibility is important because our health depends upon our circulation. No matter how well you eat, if you do not have good circulation, the delivery of oxygen and nutrients to every area of your body is poor. Circulation is critical.

So how can you achieve optimal circulation? The heart pumps blood through arteries and smaller vessels out to remote cells. In between the arteries and veins is a capillary network. Capillaries are tiny blood vessels that interlink to form networks. Capillary density is essential for adequate delivery of oxygen and nutrients to cells throughout the entire body. If you do <u>not</u> have good capillary density, you will have a problem with blood circulation.

Capillaries are extended to the parts of the body that are regularly used. If a part of the body is not used, capillaries can shrink and diminish. Imagine how poor a sedentary individual's circulation is without regular stretching. On the other hand, if an individual stretches regularly, there should be an abundance of capillary density throughout the body.

Capillaries do not extend and grow by themselves. The protein-based chemical released by the human gene to grow blood vessels is called Angiogenin. **Some scientists and Doctors say that stretching could be the key to stimulating Angiogenesis, the growth of new blood capillaries**.

Therapeutic Relief

The many benefits of stretching have become increasingly clear, such as decreases in levels of stress and anxiety, brain wave changes, decreases in heart rates and increased immune system function. However, stretching is still considered to primarily be no more than a tool to increase flexibility. The full potential of stretching has not yet been fully accepted.

Scientists are discovering more concrete evidence about the benefits of stretching. These benefits include reduced pain for individuals with arthritis; improved breathing for asthma sufferers; and increased natural killer cell activity in the immune system.

Stretching stimulates the PSNS into a state of relaxation and floor stretching also affects pressure receptors on the skin. Stress and anxiety levels, both psychological and biochemical, can be reduced through stretching. An individual can experience a more attentive, relaxed state after participating in a long stretch.

Static stretching exercises are also a form of self-massage, inasmuch as limbs are pressing against the floor and up against each other. This pressure on the skin stimulates pressure receptors.

Doctors Melzack and Wall formulated the 'gate control theory' of pain to explain why pressure stimulation alleviates pain. Pressure receptors can transmit information to the brain faster and more effectively than pain receptors due to the nerve fibres being longer and more insulated. The essence of gate control theory is that the message sent from the pressure receptors beats the message sent from pain receptors; this closes a gate in the spinal cord, which blocks the pain message.

Chronic stress is a source of pain, and stretching can be used as an effective therapy for stress relief. Stress created from our fast-moving, ever demanding lifestyles can cause muscular tension and this can quickly lead to cardiovascular problems. When we are under stress, our heart rate increases. This elevates blood pressure and stress hormone levels also rise, (e.g. norepinephrine and cortisol). At the same time, our blood flow to the immune system and digestive tract is reduced. Stretching can help to reduce muscular tension and alleviate stress.

The Medical Community

Stretching programmes are gaining more attention in the medical community. In a recent report from Florida State University, Dr. Richard Usatine, Associate Dean of medical education at the FSU College, stated that stretching can be as important as any medication, and stretching programmes may become a regular part of medicine in the future.

In Summary:

- Flexibility is important because our health fundamentally depends upon our circulation - it is now well proven that the more flexible we are, the better our circulation will be.

- Our modern, sedentary lifestyles tend to shorten and cramp our joints and muscles, leading to short term aches and pains and longer term deterioration of the nervous system.

- Yoga-type stretching is the great "missing link" in the quest to build a healthy body which will remain vigorous and active well into later life.

Chapter References

1. Alter MJ. Science of flexibility. Second Edition. Champaign, IL: Human Kinetics; 1996.

2. Chaitow L: Muscle Energy Techniques. New York, Churchill Livingstone, 1997.

3. Liebension C. Integrating rehabilitation into chiropractic practice (blending active and passive care). Chapter 2. In Liebenson C (ed.). Rehabilitation of the Spine. Baltimore, Williams and Wilkins, 1996.

4. Gossman MR, Sahrman SA, Rose SJ. Review of length-associated changes in muscle: experimental evidence and clinical implications. Phys Ther 1982; 62:1799-1808.

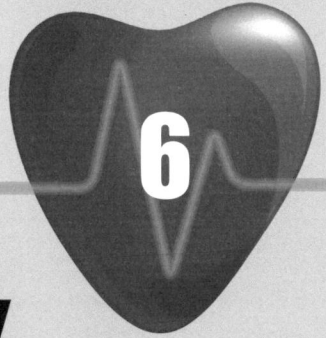

WHY
EXERCISE?

To Prevent or Reverse
Weight Gain & Obesity

Why Exercise? - To Prevent or Reverse Weight Gain & Obesity

Understanding Obesity

Obesity is basically a condition in which there is an accumulation of excess body fat on a person. A person is considered obese if he or she weighs more than 20 pounds above their maximum healthy weight (which is usually determined by height). To calculate a healthy weight and obesity, BMI (body-mass index) was generally used. More recently, waist-to-hip-ratio for men and women, not body-mass index (BMI) has been found as a more accurate measure that relates closest to increased risk of death from obesity. However, a BMI of more than 30 is still an accurate measure and considered obese. The term obesity generally refers to the overfat condition that, without doubt, increases the risk of disease.

UK Statistics on Obesity

In the UK, more than 50 percent of the adult population is obese, and many children and teenagers are now overweight or obese. Obesity statistics are at epidemic proportions and climbing, which is dramatically contributing to the rise of diabetes and cardiovascular disease. [1, 2, 3, 4] The World Health Organization and the Obesity Task Force have declared obesity as a global epidemic. [5]

Adults

- The World Health Organisation Report 2002 estimates that over 7% of all disease burden in developed countries is caused by raised BMI. [6]

- Overweight and obesity are increasing rapidly. The percentage of obese adults in England has increased by over 50% since 1996. [6]

- The WHO SURF Report 2 shows UK rates are amongst the highest in Europe. [6]

- The UK currently has the eighth highest obesity rate in the world. [7]

- In England, around 44% of men and 35% of women are overweight. [6]

- An additional 23% of men and 24% of women are obese. [6]
- Overweight and obesity increases with age, peaking in those aged 55-64. [6]
- 31% of men and 38% of women aged 16-24 are overweight or obese. [6]
- 78% of men and 70% of women aged 55-64 are overweight or obese. [6]
- Black Africans, Indians, Pakistanis, Bangladeshis and Chinese men are 4 times less likely to be obese but have similar raised waist-to-hip-ratios compared to the general population. [6]

Children

- Classification of overweight and obesity in children and adolescents is more problematic than in adults due to growth patterns and gender. The International Obesity Taskforce's new classification estimates 22% of boys and 28% of girls aged 2-15 are either overweight or obese. 6% of boys and 7% of girls are obese. [6]
- Between 1995-2005, obesity in boys aged 2-15 doubled from 3% to 6%.
- In girls of the same age, it rose from 5% to 8%. [6]

Symptoms of Obesity

The clear symptom of obesity is an accumulation of excess body fat on a person.

What does Obesity generally lead to?

Obesity puts a strain on organs and joints and an abundance of health problems are associated with obesity. **The 'obese syndrome' is linked to: glucose intolerance, insulin resistance, type 2 diabetes, hypertension, increased coronary heart disease, arthritis, cancer, and even Alzheimer's disease.** [7]

Increased risk of early death is associated with obesity. [8, 9, 10]

Why does it happen?

Research suggests that obesity results from a complex interaction of factors: genetic, environmental, metabolic, physiological, behavioural, social and racial influences. [11, 12, 13, 14, 15] However, in my experience

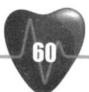

of training individuals, obesity is usually just down to a simple lack of exercise, poor eating habits and general laziness. Sadly though, if a child has obese parents, the child's risk of obesity in adulthood is two to three times that of children with normal-weight parents. [16] However, generally, obesity occurs due to overeating or poor diet, a lack of exercise, and/or a sedentary lifestyle.

Why Exercise?

Scientific Research on Obesity & Exercise

A study by a researcher at the UCLA/RAND Managed Care Centre for Psychiatric Disorders in Santa Monica, California confirmed that obesity and being overweight have serious consequences. Roland Sturm, the author of this study, found that obesity was linked to health complications including diabetes, arthritis, heart disease, strokes and certain cancers. He said, "Obesity is associated with a lot of chronic conditions, which have a large impact on health costs."

Sturm stated that our lifestyles today, such as spending more time in front of television and computers, becoming a car-obsessed culture and taking less physical activity, is the significant cause of the world's growing obesity problem.

A sedentary lifestyle consistently emerges as the important factor with obesity and weight gain in children, adolescents and adults. Excess weight gain runs in parallel with reduced physical activity. [17, 18, 19, 20, 21] In scientific studies excess fat levels relate directly to the number of hours spent watching television, working with computers or playing video games among children, adolescents, and adults. [22, 23] These activities, if minimised, could enable children and adults to lose weight. [24, 25]

Scientific research confirms that regular physical exercise along with healthy eating habits is more effective than long-term, low calorie dieting or calorie restriction. [26, 27] I personally never encourage dieting or calorie restriction, I recommend eating a healthy, balanced, nutrient-rich diet to all my clients, and to exercise six days a week!

Regular exercise is effective for obese individuals wanting to lose body fat. [28] Adolescent males who exercise have less abdominal fat than sedentary males. [29] Adding exercise to a weight loss programme

significantly improves fat loss. [30, 31, 32, 33]

For both men and women, excess fat and obesity increases the risk for heart disease, insulin resistance, type 2 diabetes, endometrial cancer, hypertension and atherosclerosis. [34] However, new research shows that it is more specifically waist-to-hip-ratio for men and women, not body-mass index (BMI) that relates closest to increased risk of death from disease in adults. [35, 36, 37, 38] Canadian researchers concluded that waist-to-hip ratio is a stronger indicator in predicting the risk of a heart attack than body mass index, (BMI). Basically, **if your waist size is dramatically larger than your hip size, you raise your risk from death from a chronic degenerative disease dramatically**.

Dr. Salim Yusuf, Director of the Population Research Institute at McMaster University and Hamilton Health Sciences, studied more than 27,000 people from 52 countries. Yusuf found that **people who had a larger waist-size, (a higher amount of abdominal fat) had a much greater risk of a heart attack. This result was consistent in men and women, across all ages, and in all regions of the world. The authors of the study concluded that a higher waist-to-hip ratio increased the chance of a heart attack three-fold**.

For children and adolescents, obesity is linked to numerous serious health issues including higher blood cholesterol, higher blood pressure and even increased left ventricular wall thickness. [39, 40]

In addition, overweight children tend to become overweight adults with increased risk of hypertension and heart disease. **The huge rise in child obesity requires immediate interventions to prevent the early death of these children**.

Scientific studies show that to successfully lose weight, obese individuals should adopt long-term goals, develop personal discipline and restructure eating and exercise behaviours. [41] Individuals with social ties or family members who are also participating in the exercise/ diet programme seem to be more successful than those who exercise and diet alone. [42] This is especially important as exercise and healthy eating proves to be the ideal combination for body fat loss, rather than either exercise or diet alone. [43, 44, 45, 46, 47]

In Summary:

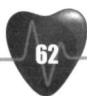

- Obesity is becoming a worldwide epidemic. If you are overweight you are greatly increasing the risk that you will suffer from one or more serious and degenerative health problems, such as diabetes, cardiovascular disease and certain types of cancer.

- If you need to lose weight, you MUST combine a healthy diet with a regular exercise routine that combines aerobic, anaerobic and resistance training for optimum health and longevity.

Chapter References

1. Lappalainen R, et al. Recent body-weight changes and weight loss practices in the European Union. Public Health Nutr 1999;2(1A):135.

2. Popkin BM, Doak CM. The obesity epidemic is a worldwide phenomenon. Nutr Rev 1998;56:106.

3. Wardle J, Griffith J. Socioeconomic status and weight control practices in British adults. J Epidemiol Community Health 2001;55:195.

4. Zimmerman MB, et al. A national study of the prevalence of over-weight and obesity in 6-12 y-old Swiss children: body mass index, body-weight perceptions and goals. Eur J Clin Nutr 2000;54:568.

5. Segal KR, et al. Body composition, not body weight, is related to cardiovascular disease risk factors and sex hormone levels in man. J Clin Invest 1987;80:1050.

6 Allender, S., Peto, V., Scarborough, P., Boxer, A., Rayner, M. (2006) Coronary Heart Disease Statistics. British Heart Foundation, London.

7 Arthritis Research Campaign. Available from http://www.arc.org.uk/ [cited 10th July 2007]

8. Taubes G. As obesity rates rise, experts struggle to explain why. Science 1998;280:1367.

9. Bender R, et al. Effect of age on excess mortality in obesity. JAMA 1999;281:1498.

10. Calle EE, et al. Body-mass index and mortality in a prospective cohort of U.S. adults. N Engl J Med 1999;341:1097.

11. Must A, et al. The disease burden associated with overweight and obesity. JAMA 1999;282:1523.

12. Carpenter WH et al. Total daily energy expenditure in free-living older African-Americans and Caucasians. Am J Physiol (Endocrinol Metab) 1998;274:E96-101.

13. Grundy SM. Multifactorial causation of obesity; implications for prevention. Am J Clin Nutr 1998;67(suppl):563S.

14. Lindroos AK, et al. Familial predisposition for obesity may modify the predictive value of serum leptin concentrations for long-term weight change in obese women. Am J Clin Nutr 1998;67:1119.

15. Rosenbaum, M, et al. Obesity. N Engl J Med 1997;337:396.

16. Zhang Y, et al. Positional cloning of the mouse obese gene and its human homologue. Nature 1994;372:425.

17. Whitaker RC, et al. Predicting obesity in young adulthood from childhood and parental obesity. N Engl J Med 1997;337:869.

18. Bar-Or O, et al. Physical activity, genetic and nutritional considerations in childhood weight management. Med Sci Sports Exerc 1998;30:2.

19. Epstein LH, et al. Exercise in treating obesity in children and adolescents. Med Sci Sports Exerc 1996;28:428.

20. Melby CL, et al. Exercise, macronutrient balance, and weight regulation. In: Lamb DR, Murray R, eds. Perspectives in exercise and sports medicine, vol. II: Exercise, nutrition, and weight control. Carmel, IN: Cooper Publishing, 1998.

21. Raitakari OT, et al. Associations between physical activity and risk factors for coronary heart disease; the Cardiovascular Risk in Young Finns Study. Med Sci Sports Exerc 1997;29:1055.

22. Ross R, et al. Exercise alone is an effective strategy for reducing obesity and related comorbidities. Exer Sport Sci Rev 2000;28:165.

23. Anderson RE, et al. Relationship of physical activity and television watching with body weight and level of fatness among children. JAMA 1998;279:938.

24. Gordon-Larsen P, et al. Adolescent physical inactivity vary by ethnicity: the National Longitudinal Study of Adolescent Health. J Pediatr 1999:135:301.

25. Gordon-Larsen P, et al. Adolescent physical activity and inactivity vary by ethnicity: the National Longitudinal Study of Adolescent Health. J Pediatr 1999;135:301.

26. Robinson TN. Reducing children's television viewing to prevent obesity: a randomized clinical trial. JAMA 1999;282:1562.

27. Bungard LB, et al. Energy requirements of middle-aged men are modifiable by physical activity. Am J Clin Nutr 1998;69:1136.

28. Klem ML, et al. A descriptive study of individuals successful at long-term maintenance of substantial weight loss. Am J Clin Nutr 1997;66:239.

29. Ross R, et al. Exercise alone is an effective strategy for reducing obesity and related comorbidities. Exer Sport Sci Rev 2000;28:165.

30. Dionne I, et al. The association between vigorous physical activities and fat deposition in male adolescents. Med Sci Sports Exerc 2000;32:392.

31. Ballor DL, Keesey RE. A meta-analysis of the factors affecting changes in body mass, fat mass and fat-free mass in males and females. Int J Obes 1991;15:717.

32. Konstantin NP, et al. Effects of dieting and exercise on fat-free body mass, oxygen uptake, and strength. Med Sci Sports Exerc 1985;17:446.

33. Kraemer WJ, et al. Compatibility of high-intensity strength and endurance training on hormonal and skeletal muscle adaptations. J Appl Physiol 1995;78:976.

34. McMurray RG, et al. Responses of endurance trained subjects to caloric deficits induced by diet or exercise. Med Sci Sports Exerc 1985;17:574.

35. Hunter GR, et al. Fat distribution, physical activity, and cardiovascular risk factors. Med Sci Sports Exerc 1997;29:362.

36. Després J-P. Visceral obesity, insulin resistance, and dyslipidemia: contribution of endurance exercise training to the treatment of the plurimetabolic syndrome. Exerc Sport Sci Rev 1997;25:271.

37. Folsom R, et al. Body fat distribution and 5-year risk of death in older women. JAMA 1993;269:483.

38. Rexrode KM, et al. Abdominal adiposity and coronary heart disease in women. JAMA 1998;280:1843.

39. Williams MJ, et al. Regional fat distribution in women and risk of cardiovascular disease. Am J Clin Nutr 1997;65:855.

40. Daniels SR, et al. Body fat distribution and cardiovascular risk factors in children. Circulation 1999;99:541.

41. Freedman DS, et al. Relation of circumferences and skinfold thicknesses to lipid and insulin concentrations in children and adolescents: the Bogalusa Heart Study. Am J Clin Nutr 1999;69:308.

42. McArdle WD, Toner MM. Application of exercise for weight control: the exercise prescription. In: Frankle RT, Yang M-U, eds. Obesity and weight control. Rockville, MD: Aspen, 1988.

43. Wing RR, et al. Benefits of recruiting participants with friends and increasing social support for weight loss and maintenance. J Consult Clin Psychol 1999;67:132.

44. Ebbeling CB, Rodriguez NR. Effect of exercise combined with diet therapy on protein utilization in obese children. Med Sci Sports Exerc 1999;31:378.

45. National Institutes of Health, National Heart, Lung, and blood institute. Obesity evaluation initiative, Clinical guidelines and the identification, evaluation, and treatment of overweight and obesity in adults. Bethesda, MD: National Institutes of Health, June, 1998.

46. Racette SB, et al. Effects of aerobic exercise and dietary carbohydrate on

energy expenditure and body composition during weight reduction in obese women. Am J Clin Nutr 1995;61:486.

47. Waddem TA. Characteristic of successful weight loss maintenance. In: Pi-Sunyer FX, Allison DB, eds. Obesity treatment: establishing goals, improving outcomes, and establishing the research agenda. New York: Plenum, 1995.

48. Wimore JH. Increasing physical activity: alterations in body mass and composition. Am J Clin Nutr 1996;63(suppl):456S.

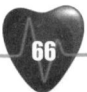

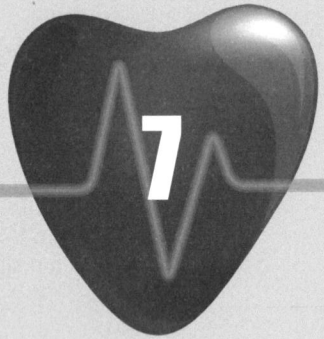

WHY EXERCISE?

To Prevent Cardiovascular Disease

Why Exercise? - to Prevent Cardiovascular Disease

Understanding Cardiovascular Disease

The heart and vascular system is one of the most important systems in the body. Its primary function is to deliver oxygen and vital nutrients to cells throughout the body. The human heart pumps 2,500 - 5,000 gallons of blood through approximately 60,000 miles of blood vessels everyday. We need to look after this system. We need to look after our hearts.

Cardiovascular disease is a term used to describe a variety of dysfunctional conditions of the heart, arteries and veins. These conditions include angina, heart attack, diseases of the heart muscle or valves, heart failure, stroke, and pain from poor blood flow to the legs.

UK Statistics on Cardiovascular Disease (CVD)

Cardiovascular disease is the leading cause of death in all industrialised nations.

Mortality rates:

- 37% of people die from CVD. [1]
- 49% of this 37% die from Coronary Heart Disease (CHD) (1 in 5 of all men, 1 in 6 of all women).
- CHD caused 105,000 deaths in 2004 in the UK.
- CHD is the most common cause of premature death in the UK (death before 75).
- 28% of these 37% die from a stroke.
- Death rates from CVD and CHD have been falling in the UK since the early 1970s. [1]
- For people under 75, CVD deaths have fallen by 38% and CHD deaths have fallen by 44% since 1996, fastest in those aged 55 and over, slowest in younger age groups. [1]
- 58% of this decline is attributed to reductions in major risk factors such as smoking. [1]

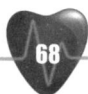

- UK-based South Asians (Indians, Bangladeshis, Pakistanis and Sri Lankans) have a higher than average mortality from CHD (46% higher for men, 51% higher for women). [1]

- UK-based Caribbeans and West Africans have lower than average mortality rates from CHD (around half that of the UK population as a whole for men, and 2/3rds of the rate for women). [1]

Morbidity rates

- The incidence of heart attack in men aged between 30 and 69 is 0.6% and 0.2% in women. This increases with age. Based on this, there are around 55,000 heart attacks each year in men under 75 living in the UK and 20,000 in women. [1]

- The Health Survey for England suggests the prevalence of CVD in England is 7.4% in men and 4.5% in women. [1]

- Overall the British Heart Foundation estimates there to be just over 1.5 million men living in the UK who have had CVD and about 1.1 million women. [1]

- **In 2004, CVD was the 2nd most commonly reported longstanding illness in Great Britain** (after musculoskeletal conditions). [1]

Symptoms of Cardiovascular Disease

Cardiovascular conditions may often exist without symptoms, which means they can often go untreated. When symptoms appear, such as pain in a poor-circulation area, the extent and variety of the symptoms usually depends on the extent to which the normal blood flow is interrupted. With severe blood flow interruption, many symptoms can occur.

Signs of severe blood flow interruption include:

- Chest discomfort or pain

- Sweating

- Nausea

- Shortness of breath

- Faintness

What does Cardiovascular Disease generally lead to?

Because symptoms often go unnoticed and untreated until late in the disease process, serious health issues often occur. These conditions include heart attack, stroke, kidney damage and even death. As mentioned, **CVD is the leading cause of death in all industrialised nations**.

Why Does it Happen?

Diseases of the heart become more common with age in industrialised nations. Modern industrialisation tends to create sedentary lifestyles. **People who are sedentary have twice the risk of heart disease as those who are physically active**.

Statistics prove that men have a greater risk of heart attacks than women.

Controllable risk factors include:

- Stress

- Alcohol consumption

- Smoking

- Poor diet

- High blood pressure

- Diabetes

- Lack of exercise

- Obesity or weight problems

Why Exercise?

Scientific Research on Cardiovascular Disease & Exercise

Hypertension (high blood pressure) is a primary risk factor for CVD. The risk for hypertension is generally higher in men than in women, and naturally rises with age. However, exercise training can be used as an effective means to prevent and treat hypertension. [2, 3, 4, 5, 6, 7, 8]

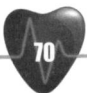

Unfortunately, a brisk walking programme may not provide satisfactory stimulus to reduce hypertension. [9] **Regular aerobic exercise however, can help control the tendency for blood pressure to increase over time and with age**. [10]

Over time, patients with mild hypertension benefit from the effects of aerobic exercise training. [11, 12, 13, 14, 15] In fact, middle-aged men with mild hypertension significantly benefit from 6 months of regular aerobic exercise. [16] In addition, older hypertensive men and women significantly benefit from 9 months of low-intensity, aerobic exercise. [17]

Although the precise mechanisms for how exercise training lowers blood pressure remains unknown, there are some theories.

Contributing factors of exercise that may lower blood pressure are:

• Capillary/small blood vessel growth (angiogenesis).

• Reduced sympathetic nervous system activity following exercise training (lowered stress levels). [3, 18, 19, 20]

To manage hypertension, regular aerobic exercise and proper diet can help. These habits help maintain healthy body weight, which is an important criterion for the maintenance of good blood pressure. [11, 4, 21, 22] **Even when aerobic training does not lower high blood pressure, it does lower the mortality rate of the condition**. [23]

One important caution to note is that resistance training is less effective at lowering blood pressure than aerobic exercise training. [10, 24, 25, 26, 27, 28] Regular aerobic exercise contributes to enhanced function and symptomatic improvements in cardiovascular function. [29, 30]

Aerobic exercise is an important, effective, protective means to improve cardiovascular functional capacity. As a result, exercise helps individuals avoid heart disease. [31]

For long-term health, a programme should be based on activities that are proven by exercise science to be ultimately healthy. In addition, the programme should include behavioural objectives that will improve the individual's compliance and encourage the accomplishment of individual goals. [32]

The most effective exercise programmes for CVD prevention and treatment focus on individual needs, and use low-to-moderate levels of aerobic exercise intensity, rather than intense physical activity. The prescribed exercises in heart-healthy programmes use rhythmic, big-muscle movements that stimulate the cardiovascular system effectively. [33, 34, 35, 36]

For cardiac rehabilitation, a comprehensive exercise programme should focus on improving a patient's longevity and quality of life. It should also centre on reducing the individual's risk for mortality. [31, 37, 38] When resistance training exercises are implemented into a cardiac rehabilitation program, they restore strength, mental outlook and quality of life. [39, 40, 41]

Even for adults with advanced heart disease up to age 65, no adverse effects have been reported from resistance training performed at low-to-moderate intensity levels. [42] And although data is limited, even heart transplant patients respond positively to aerobic exercise training. [43, 44, 45]

Jing Fang, M.D. and colleagues from the Albert Einstein College of Medicine in the Bronx, New York, say that **exercise may do more to ward off death from heart disease than reducing calorie intake**. This determination comes from a 17-year study of almost 9,800 individuals.

The study, funded by the US government, appeared in the American Journal of Preventive Medicine also said "**Expending physical energy through physical activity may be the key to cutting the risks of heart disease and living a longer, healthier life**" Fang says. "Exercise offers the most productive behavioural strategy by which to extend healthy life," she adds.

Another study was based on data from 9,611 adults in their 50s and 60s. It showed that those who exercised were about 35 - 45% less likely to die in the next eight years than those who lived sedentary lifestyles. The results were published in the Journal of Medicine and Science in Sports and Exercise recently.

The article was based on a study by researchers at the University of Michigan Medical School and the VA Ann Arbor Healthcare System. The lead author, Caroline Richardson, M.D., Assistant Professor of

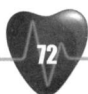

Family Medicine, said, "Everyone received a benefit from exercising." She also said that the measurable results were conclusive.

As people age (particularly women after menopause), if they do <u>not</u> exercise, they lose their artery elasticity. This causes high blood pressure and enlarges the heart. But a 12-week study involving a group of 14 women, all around 60 years of age (who did not exercise before the study but were otherwise healthy) showed **elasticity of arteries can be improved by nearly 50 percent through regular exercise**.

This study was lead by Kerrie Moreau, PhD, from the University of Colorado Human Cardiovascular Research Laboratory in Boulder, CO. She presented the study at the Experimental Biology meeting in 2002. The authors concluded that the marked improvement in artery elasticity in such a short time could make a big difference in reducing the risk of heart disease.

In another study by Dr. Barry A. Franklin, Director of Cardiac Rehabilitation at William Beaumont Hospital in Royal Oak, Michigan, Franklin found that **resistance training improves body composition and cardiovascular function**. Dr. Franklin says, "**When muscles are stronger, heart rate and blood pressure become lower**."

Dr. Timothy Wessel, from the University of Florida Medical School, performed a study of more than 900 women. His results were published in the Journal of the American Medical Association. The findings showed that, "**lack of physical fitness is a stronger risk factor for developing heart disease then being overweight or obese**."

In another study from the University of Pisa, more specific findings have been revealed. **Blood vessels of older people who exercised regularly functioned as well as those of athletes less than half their age**.

The Pisa study, published in the Journal of Circulation was written by Dr. Stefano Taddei. Taddei explained that one effect of ageing is a reduction in a mechanism within blood cells that causes nitrous oxide to be released. This mechanism diminishes its efficiency as we age. Nitrous oxide protects arteries and veins against clogging and also assists in dilating the vessels when the heart needs more blood. But Dr. Taddei's studies concluded that **individuals who performed moderate levels of regular exercise five days a week (rather than intensive training)**

dramatically improved the function of their blood vessels.

Another study was presented at the American Heart Association's Sixth Annual Conference on Arteriosclerosis. This study was led by author Kunihiko Aizawa, M.Sc., a Ph.D. candidate at the University of Western Ontario. Aizawa found that a lifestyle management programme of diet and exercise improves the health of vasculature. Therefore, according to the researchers, it may also reduce the risk of high blood pressure, diabetes, heart attacks and stroke.

Deborah R. Young MD, Assistant Professor at the John Hopkins University School of Medicine in Baltimore, studied Tai Chi's effects on the heart. Young determined that Tai Chi lowers blood pressure in older adults nearly as much as moderate-intensity aerobic exercise.

Young presented at the American Heart Association's Epidemiology and Prevention Conference. She said, "**It could be that for elderly people, just getting up and doing some slow, balancing movements could reduce high blood pressure**."

Stroke

Understanding a Stroke

A stroke is a sudden disruption in blood flow to the brain, which can cause damage to a part of the brain where the blood flow disruption occurs. Over half of all strokes are caused when a blood clot forms in an artery in the brain, called cerebral thrombosis. Another major cause is when a fragment of a blood clot forms in another part of the body, then travels in the blood. This clot then lodges in an artery supplying the brain with blood. This process is termed a cerebral embolism. A cerebral hemorrhage is another major cause of stroke. This occurs when an artery supplying the brain ruptures and blood seeps out into the surrounding tissues.

UK Statistics on Stroke

- Around 130,000 people in the UK have a first stroke every year - about one person every five minutes. [46]

- Stroke can affect people of any age. Nine out of ten strokes occur in people over the age of 55. [46]

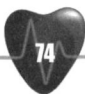

- Men are more often affected than women. People from Asian, African, and Afro-Caribbean backgrounds are more at risk. [46]

- High blood pressure, smoking, diabetes, a previous mini-stroke, binge drinking/eating, and having someone else in the family who has had a stroke increase the risk of a person suffering a stroke. [46]

- Stroke is the commonest cause of severe disability and is often fatal. [46]

- Every year, an estimated 150,000 people in the UK have a stroke. Most people affected are over 65, but anyone can have a stroke, including children and even babies. [47]

- A stroke is the third most common cause of death in the UK. It is also the single most common cause of severe disability. More than 250,000 people live with disabilities caused by stroke. [47]

Shocking research confirms an estimated 15 million people worldwide survive a stroke each year.

The initial after-effects of a stroke will depend predominantly on the location and the extent of the tissue damage in the brain as a result of the stroke. Almost one–third of all individuals who experience a stroke make a full recovery.

Common symptoms that can be overcome are: a weakness on one side of the body; an inability to move one side of the body; a loss of control of intricate or large movements; difficulty in maintaining balance, and difficulty in understanding what others are saying.

Blood clots and ruptured blood vessels are much more likely to form in arteries that have been damaged by atherosclerosis. Atherosclerosis is the hardening of arteries, caused by fatty deposits that build up in artery walls. These deposits reduce the diameter of blood vessels and cause blood pressure to rise. High blood pressure is the number 1 cause of a stroke.

Why Exercise?

Scientific Research on Stroke & Exercise
Just as regular exercise can reduce the risk of a heart attack, physical activity may also help prevent stroke. The Prevention Advisory Board of

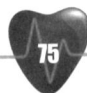

the National Stroke Association (NSA) recommends taking "a brisk walk for 30 minutes a day" as one of 10 strategies to help prevent a stroke. By preventing a stroke, the incidence of adult disability will greatly diminish, as stroke is a leading cause of adult disability.

Philip B. Gorelick is Professor of Neurology at Chicago's Rush Hospital and Chairman of the NSA panel. Gorelick says that **exercise is so important to cardiovascular health in general, we now have the evidence to say that physical activity is an important factor to protect against stroke**.

In Summary:

- **Looking after the heart and circulatory system is fundamental to good health, yet cardiovascular disease is at an all time high as a result of our modern way of life, poor diet and failure to take adequate exercise.**

- **Improving your circulation by regular aerobic exercise is a key insurance against the threats to health represented by high blood pressure which, if left unchecked, often triggers cardiovascular disease and stroke.**

- **As we have already seen in Chapter 5, improved circulation also provides many other health benefits by strengthening the immune system, thus forming a first line defence against many serious diseases. It also increases vitality and longevity - so you'll enjoy life for longer!**

Chapter References

1 Allender, S., Peto, V., Scarborough, P., Boxer, A., Rayner, M. (2006) Coronary Heart Disease Statistics. British Heart Foundation, London.

2. Baglivo HP, et al. Effect of moderate physical training on left ventricular mass in mild hypertensive persons. Hypertension 1990;15(Suppl.I):1.

3. Dengel DR, et al. Improvements in blood pressure, glucose metabolism, and lipoprotein lipids after aerobic exercise plus weight loss in obese, hypertensive middle-aged men. Metabolism 1998;47:1075.

4. Hagberg JM. Physical activity, physical fitness, and blood pressure. In: Leon

A, ed. Physical activity and cardiovascular health. Champaign, IL: Human Kinetics, 1997.

5. Kraemer WJ, et al. Resistance training combined with bench-step aerobics enhances women's health profile. Med Sci Sports Exerc 2001;33:259.

6. O'Conner PJ, et al. State anxiety and ambulatory blood pressure following resistance exercise in females. Med Sci Sports Exerc 1993;25:516.

7. Urata H, et al. Antihypertensive and volume-depleting effects of mild exercise on essential hypertension. Hypertension 1987;9:245.

8. Wilmore JH, et al. Heart rate and blood pressure changes with endurance training: The Heritage Family Study. Med Sci Sports Exerc 2001;33:107.

9. Cooper AR, et al. What is the magnitude of blood pressure response to a programme of moderate intensity exercise? Randomised controlled trail among sedentary adults with unmedicated hypertension. Br J Gen Pract 2000 ec;50:958.

10. Paffenbarger RS Jr, et al. Physical activity and hypertension: an epidemiological view. Ann Med 1991;23:19.

11. American College of Sports Medicine. Position Stand. Physical activity, physical fitness, and hypertension. Med Sci Sports Exerc 1993;25:i.

12. Coconie CC, et al. Effect of exercise training on blood pressure in 70 to 79 year old men and women. Med Sci Sports Exerc 1991;23:505.

13. Hagberg JM, et al. Effects of exercise training on 60 to 69 year old persons with essential hypertension. Am J Cardiol 1989;64:348.

14. Kohno K, et al. Depressor effect by exercise training is associated with amelioration of hyperinsulinemia and sympathetic overactivity. Intern Med 2000;39:1013.

15. Nho H, et al. Exercise training in female patients with a family history of hypertension. Eur J Appl Physiol 1998;78:1.

16. Choquette G. Ferguson RJ. Blood pressure reduction in "borderline" hypertensives following physical training. Can Med Assoc J:1973;108:699.

17. Hagberg JM, et al. Effects of exercise training on 60 to 69 year old persons with essential hypertension. Am J Cardiol 1989;64:348.

18. Amaral SL, et al. Exercise training normalizes wall-to-lumen ratio of the gracilis muscle arterioles and reduces pressure in spontaneously hypertensive rats. J Hypertens 2000;18:1563.

19. Fagard RH. Tipton CM. Physical activity, fitness, and hypertension. In: Bouchard C, et al., eds. Physical activity, fitness and health. Champaign, IL: Human Kinetics, 1994.

20. O' Sullivan SE, Bell C. The effects of exercise and training on human cardiovascular reflex control. J Auton Nerv Syst 2000 3;81:16.

21. Kelemen MH. Exercise training combined with antihypertensive drug therapy: effects on lipids, blood pressure, and left ventricular mass. JAMA 1990;263:2766.

22. Stevens VJ, et al. Long-term weight loss and changes in blood pressure: results of the Trials of Hypertensive Prevention, phase II. Ann Intern Med 2001 2;134:1.

23. Blair SN, et al. Physical fitness and all-cause mortality: a prospective study of healthy men and women. JAMA 1989;262:2395.

24. Hagberg JM, et al. Effect of weight training on blood pressure and hemodynamics in hypertensive adolescents. J Pediatr 104:147, 1984.

25. Wiley RL, et al. Isometric exercise training lowers resting blood pressure. Med Sci Sports Exerc 1992;24:749.

26. Kelly G. Dynamic resistance exercise and resting blood pressure in adults: A meta analysis. J Appl Physiol 1997;82:1559.

27. Kelley GA, Kelley KS. Progressive resistance exercise and resting blood pressure: A meta-analysis of randomized controlled trials. Hypertension. 2000;35:838.

28. Orbach P, Lowenthal DT. Evaluation and treatment of hypertension in active individuals. Med Sci Sports Exerc 1998;30(suppl):S354.

29. Mairana A, et al. Effect of aerobic and resistance exercise training on vascular function in heart disease. Am J Physiol Heart Circ Physiol 2000;279: H1999-.

30. Meyer K. Exercise training in heart failure: recommendations based on current research. Med Sci Sports Exerc 2001;33:525.

31. Shephard RJ, Baldy GJ. Exercise as cardiovascular therapy. Circulation 1999;99:963.

32. Franklin BA, et al. ACSM's guidelines for exercise testing and prescription. 6th ed. Balitmore: Lippincott Williams & Wilkins, 2000.

33. Matsusaki M, et al. influence of workload on the antihypertensive effect of exercise. Clin Exp Pharmacol Physiol 1992;19:471.

34. Ahmaidi S et al. Effects of interval training at the ventilatory threshold on clinical and cardiorespiratory responses in elderly humans. Eur J Appl Physiol 1998;78:170.

35. Meyer K. Exercise training in heart failure: recommendations based on current research. Med Sci Sports Exerc 2001;33:525.

36. Meyer K, et al. Interval training in patients with severe chronic heart failure: analysis and recommendations for exercise procedures. Med Sci Sports Exerc 1997;29:306.

37. Oldridge NB, et al. Cardiac rehabilitation after myocardial infarction:

combined experience of randomized clinical trials. JAMA 1998;260:945.

38. Engebretson TO, et al. Quality of life and anxiety in a phase II cardiac rehabilitation program. Med Sci Sports Exerc 1999;31:216.

39. Fardy PS, Yanowitz FG. Cardiac rehabilitation, adult fitness, and exercise testing, Baltimore: Williams & Wilkins, 1996.

40. McCartney N. Role of resistance training in heart disease. Med Sci Sports Exerc 1998;30 (suppl):S396.

41. McCartney N. Acute responses to resistance and safety. Med Sci Sports Exerc 1999;31:31.

42. King ML, et al. The hemodynamic effects of isotonic exercise using hand-held weights in patients with heart failure. J Heart Lung Transplant 2000;19:1209.

43. Badenhop DT. The therapeutic role of exercise in patients with orthotopic heart transplant. Med Sci Sports Exerc 1995;27:975.

44. Braith RW. Exercise training in patients with CHF and heart transplant recipients. Med Sci Sports Exerc 1998;30(suppl):S367.

45. Keteyian S, et al. Cardiovascular reponse of heart transplant patients to exercise training. J Appl Physiol 1991;70:2627.

46 BBC December 2005 Stroke. Available from http://www.bbc.co.uk/health/conditions/stroke1.shtml [cited 11 July 2007]

47 The Stroke Association 2007 Information. Available from http://www.stroke.org.uk/information/index.html [cited 11 July 2007]

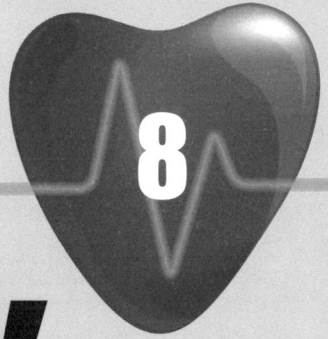

WHY
EXERCISE?
To Prevent Cancer

Why Exercise? - to Prevent Cancer

Understanding Cancer

Cancer is the uncontrolled growth of abnormal, or immature (and not fully functional) cells. These cells form abnormal cell clusters. These cell clusters become a visible mass, otherwise known as a tumour.

As cells form a clump, the cluster is called a primary tumour. But cells from a primary tumour can break away and start to grow elsewhere in the body, forming secondary tumours. This process is called metastasis. When cancer spreads to other organs, the cancer is called metastatic.

For example, liver cancer that spreads to the breast is not breast cancer; it is metastatic liver cancer. There are more than 200 different types of cancers, but four of them – breast, lung, bowel and prostate – account for over half of all new cases.

UK Statistics on Cancer

- **One in three people will be affected by cancer at some stage in their lives**. [1] Choose not to be one of them!

- There are about 200 different types of cancer affecting all the different body tissues. [2]

- In the UK in 2005, there were 153,491 deaths from cancer. [3]

- Overall, mortality from cancer is decreasing despite increasing incidence. In the 30 year period between 1976 and 2005, the age standardised mortality rates for all malignant neoplasms fell by 17% from 218 to 180 per 100,000 population. [4]

- In 2002 there were 22,504 men diagnosed with lung cancer in the UK. This works out to be 65 cases for every 100,000 men in the UK. [5] The calculated lifetime risk of lung cancer for a man in the UK is 1 in 13. [5] The age-standardised mortality rate for lung cancer has halved from 107 deaths per 100,000 men in 1971 to 53 deaths per 100,000 males in 2005. This reflects the fall in tobacco consumption in the male population since the causal link between lung cancer and tobacco smoking was established in the mid-twentieth century. There are now more female deaths from lung cancer than from any other cancer, including breast cancer. Lung cancer mortality rates for females have increased from 18

per 100,000 in 1971 to 30 per 100,000 women in 2005, thus the male:female ratio has decreased from approximately 6:1 to 7:4 over this period. [4]

- Bowel (colorectal) cancer caused over 16,000 deaths in the UK in 2005: the ratio of colon cancer to rectal cancer is 7:4.Colorectal cancer mortality rates are substantially higher in men than in women – 23 per 100,000 males compared with 14 per 100,000 females in 2005. 70% of deaths from large bowel cancer occur in people aged 70 and over. Mortality rates from colorectal cancer are falling in the UK despite increasing incidence. Between 1996 and 2005, the male age-standardised rate fell by 17% and the female rate by 20%. [4]

- Overall, prostate cancer is the most common cancer in men but other cancers are more common in younger age-groups. Prostate cancer caused 10,000 deaths in 2005. More than 85% of these deaths were in men over 70 years old. [4]

- For men aged 20-39, testicular cancer is the most common. [5]

- For testicular cancer there were 1,900 men newly diagnosed in 2002. This is a rate of 6.5 cases for every 100,000 men in the UK. [5]

- If you are looking only at cancer in children (under 15s) then leukaemia is the commonest type of cancer. [5]

- Breast Cancer: In 2002

- 41,720 women were diagnosed with breast cancer in the UK. [5]

- This works out to be just under 116 cases for every 100,000 women. [5]

- The incidence of breast cancer in Japan is much lower than in the USA or the UK. But the incidence of breast cancer in Japanese women living in the USA is the same as for the general population of American women. To doctors, **this implies that the causes of breast cancer are probably more closely related to lifestyle and the environment than they are to our genetic make up**. [5]

- Between 1996 and 2005 the number of female breast cancer deaths fell from 13,705 to 12,417 and the age-standardised mortality rate fell by nearly a fifth (18%), despite large increases in incidence. [4]

- More than half of all deaths (54%) from breast cancer are in

women aged over 70 years. Breast cancer also causes around 90 deaths in men in the UK each year. [4]

Symptoms of Cancer

Symptoms of cancer are completely dependent on the cancer site, the size of the tumour, and how it is affecting the surrounding organs or structures. If cancer is spreading, then symptoms may appear in different parts of the body. This actually makes it harder to diagnose, even though at this point, the cancer is usually quite advanced.

As cancer grows, it begins to push on nearby organs, blood vessels, and nerves. This pressure often creates some of the signs and symptoms of cancer.

Cancer often forms with no symptoms until the cancer has grown quite large. At that point, the symptoms will occur. These common symptoms include pain; fever; chronic fatigue; feeling and being sick; mouth ulcers and problems; feeling low; bowel problems; breathing problems or weight loss.

What does Cancer generally lead to?

Cancer often leads to early death. It is the cause of more than a quarter of all deaths in the UK. However, the Fred Hutchinson Cancer Research Centre (FHCRC) says that survival rates improve dramatically when cancers are diagnosed early. This is because early diagnosis catches the cancer when the disease is still confined to the organ of origin. "Early detection provides one of the most promising opportunities to reduce the incidence of advanced cancer and cancer deaths" says the FHCRC.

This organisation is the home of two Nobel Prize laureates and is an independent, non-profit research institution dedicated to the development and advancement of biomedical technology to eliminate cancer and other potentially fatal diseases, (the FHCRC receives more funding from the National Institutes of Health than any other independent U.S. research centre).

Why Does it Happen?

Environmental factors and lifestyle habits are two major contributors to the incidence of cancer. Poor lifestyle habits linked to cancer include

poor diet, **physical inactivity**, smoking, emotional stress, drinking alcohol and being overweight.

A study of nearly 50,000 twins showed that a strong family history of cancer did <u>not</u> directly relate to the development of cancer. In fact, environmental factors and lifestyle habits accounted for most of the risk, not genetic factors as previously thought by many scientists.

Douglas Easton, PhD, the author of this study and Director of the Genetic Epidemiology Unit at Strangeways Research Laboratories at Cambridge University, UK, says that **preventing cancer is clearly each person's responsibility**.

In another study, scientists studied identical twins because they have all the same genes. This study was performed with a hope of discovering if cancer is genetic or environmental. The study was conclusive, because even when one of a pair of identical twins had cancer, the other did not. In this study, Kari Hemminki, MD, PhD and Professor of Medicine, Biosciences Department, Karolinska Institute in Stockholm, Sweden, linked smoking, alcohol, diet, and physical inactivity to cancer.

In another report, Dr. Majid Ezzati, a researcher at the Harvard School of Public Health, stated that **poor diet, excess weight and a lack of physical activity are some of the main reasons people develop cancer**.

A major new review of over seven million worldwide cancer deaths in 2001 concluded that more than one-third of the incidences of cancer were a result of common environmental factors that could have been avoided. Ezzati says, "Every cancer has a genetic route, but genetic changes are the result of environment and behaviour."

Why Exercise?

Scientific Research on Cancer & Exercise

The Fred Hutchinson Cancer Research Center states, "The best way to fight cancer is to prevent it."

Carefully prescribed physical activity is essential for overall health. [6, 7] In the case of cancer, low-to-moderate exercise is an effective preventive strategy. [8, 9] A study conducted on 122,000 women showed that exercising for at least 1 hour/day reduced breast cancer risk by

20%. [10] **Increased levels of exercise significantly reduce cancer risk and mortality**. [11, 12, 13, 14, 15]

Dr. Anne McTiernan, an Internist at the FHCRC, reviewed thirty-six studies on breast cancer prevention. She reported that twenty-four of them identified exercise as a measure to protect against the disease. The studies that showed the positive effects were the groups that exercised for three to fours hours each week. The results from the other twelve groups (ones that exercised less than 3-4 hours per week) may suggest that lower levels of exercise are not enough to protect against breast cancer.

In another study on 66,568 women, McTiernan's analysis of the results suggested that **women who exercise regularly have a 22% decreased risk of breast cancer**. McTiernan also found that the lean women in the group had added protection. The increase in breast cancer for overweight women may be due to an increased amount of estrogen, which is stored in body fat, and is known to promote breast cancer growth. "**Exercise and weight-control work hand-in-hand to prevent breast cancer**," she said.

Dr. Tim Byers, Professor of Preventive Medicine at the University of Colorado School of Medicine, in Denver, is a spokesperson for the American Cancer Society. Byers says, "Reduced body fat in women who exercise is the most likely explanation for the protective effects observed in some studies." Dr. Byers also says, "**There is growing evidence to suggest that adolescent girls who exercise may have a lower risk of breast cancer later in life**."

Dennis Savaiano, Dean of Purdue's School of Consumer and Family Sciences and Professor of Food and Nutrition says, "**Poor diet and lack of exercise are behind just as many cancer cases as smoking**."

Another study relating to this topic was published in the Journal of the National Cancer Institute. The lead author was Leslie Bernstein, PhD., AFLAC Chair in Cancer Research and Professor of Preventive Medicine at the Keck School.

Bernstein found a variety of lifestyle factors that influence breast cancer risk are:

- Smoking

- Physical inactivity

- Alcohol consumption

In this study, **women who exercised regularly had a 20% lower risk of developing breast cancer than women who did not exercise**.

Breast cancer represents the leading cause of death in young women aged 25 to 44 years. [16] However, studies justify exercise to reduce the risk of contracting several forms of cancer. [9, 10, 17, 18, 19]

Also, for breast cancer survivors, exercise has proved an important measure for intervention. [16, 20, 21, 22] More and more scientific studies also support the benefits of an exercise programme for cancer patients.

The American Cancer Society recommends exercise to reduce the fatigue, loss of strength and endurance that are common side effects with chemotherapy.

The National Cancer Institute recommends light-to-moderate-intensity exercise to manage fatigue, improve physical energy, and to improve psychological outlook for people with cancer. Also, cancer patients who experience fatigue and/or a loss of bone and muscular mass benefit from regular physical activity. It can help them to return to independence and a normal lifestyle. [23, 24, 25] For cancer patients, even a home-based regular exercise programme can reduce fatigue, improve energy levels, and enhance quality of life. [26, 27, 28]

Skin cancer, or melanoma, is the most common form of cancer in humans. So many people die every year from skin cancer around the world, and this figure is rising yearly, possibly due to the deterioration of the ozone layer.

In a new study, published in the May 2006 Journal Carcinogenesis it was found that mice that exercised improved their immunity against skin cancer. Two groups were exposed to ultraviolet light. The group that had the running wheel not only developed 32 percent fewer tumours when exposed to ultraviolet B (UVB) light (which is known to cause skin cancer in humans) but the tumours developed more slowly and were smaller than in the group that could not have running wheel access. "**Exercise stimulates the death of developing cancer cells**," said the

study leader, Allan Conney of Rutgers University.

Finally, research suggests that low-to-moderate daily exercise can improve health and functional capacity in cancer patients. [16] In a study on breast cancer patients, exercise relieved depression, improved self-esteem and reduced anxiety in patients. [26]

How Exercise Fights Cancer – The Immune System

The immune system's prime function is to protect the body against infection and the development of cancer. Strengthening and enhancing the immune system is very important to achieve resistance against diseases, including cancer. Chronic infections and diseases will only occur when the immune system is weak.

Exercise immunology focuses on the interactions of environmental, physical and psychological factors with immune system function. This is a growing field in education. However, many studies to date have already confirmed that competitive high-intensity exercise increases susceptibility to illness and disease. [27] Basically, exercise can either positively or negatively affect immune system function.

Research is concluding that light-to-moderate physical exercise strengthens the immune system, which increases protection against cancer. [28, 29, 30] However, high-intensity exercise suppresses immune function and therefore, increases risk of cancer. [31, 32, 33, 34, 35, 36, 37, 38]

Moderate long-term aerobic exercise positively affects immune function in young and old individuals. [39, 40, 41] On the other hand, long-term resistance training shows no benefit toward improved immune system function. [42]

In Summary:

- **One in three of us will be affected by some form of cancer at some stage in our lives. Although the mortality rate is falling, due to improved medical techniques, the number of people affected is rising just as quickly as an inevitable result of the stress of modern living, poor diet, lack of exercise and environmental factors.**

- **Don't be a statistic! Making sensible lifestyle changes and, in**

particular, ensuring that moderate, aerobic exercise is a regular feature of your life will help regulate your weight, strengthen your immune system and consequently reduce your risk of developing cancer.

Chapter References

1. BBC Cancer. Available from http://www.bbc.co.uk/health/conditions/cancer/ [cited 10 July 2007]

2. Cancer Research UK 25 June 2007 What Causes Cancer? Available from http://www.cancerhelp.org.uk/help/default.asp?page=119 [cited 10 July 2007]

3. Cancer Research UK May 2007 Cancer Mortality Statistics. Available from http://info.cancerresearchuk.org/cancerstats/mortality/ [cited 10 July 2007]

4. Cancer Research UK May 2007 Trends in UK Cancer Mortality Statistics. Available from http://info.cancerresearchuk.org/cancerstats/mortality/ timetrends/ [cited 10 July 2007]

5. Cancer Research UK 25 June 2007 About Cancer: Cancer Statistics: Incidence, Survival and Mortality. Available from http://www.cancerhelp.org. uk/help/default.asp?page=154 [cited 10 July 2007]

6. Blair SN, et al. Physical activity, nutrition, and chronic disease. Med Sci Sports Exerc 1996;28:335.

7. Heath GW, Fentem PH. Physical activity among persons with disabilities – a public health perspective. Exerc Sport Sci Rev 1997;25:195.

8. Kramer MM, Wells CL. Does physical activity reduce risk of estrogen-dependant cancer in women? Med Sci Sports Exerc 1996;28:322.

9 Wells CL. Physical activity and cancer prevention. Focus on breast cancer. ACSM's Health Fitness J 1999;3 (1):13.

10. Rockhill B, et al. A prospective study of recreational physical activity and breast cancer risk. Arch Intern Med 1999;159:2290.

11. Hsing AW, et al. Risk factor for colorectal cancer in a prospective study among US white men, Int J Cancer 1998;77:549.

12. Lee IM, et al. Physical activity and the risk of cancer. Int J Epidemiol 1999;28:286.

13. Martinez ME, et al. Leisure-time physical activity, body size and colon cancer in women. Nurses' Health Study Research Group. J Natl Cancer Inst 1997;89:948.

14. Martinez ME, et al. Physical activity, body mass index and prostaglandin E2 levels in rectal mucosa. J Natl Cancer Inst 1999;91:950.

15. Platz EA, et al. Physical activity and benign prostatic hyperplasia. Arch Int Med 1998;158:2349.

16. Hicks JE. Exercise for cancer patients. In: Basmajian JV, Wolf SL, eds. Therapeutic exercise. 5th ed. Baltimore: Williams and Wilkins, 1990.

17. Cohn LA, et al. Voluntary exercise and experimental cancer. Adv Exp Med Biol 1992;322:41.

18. Paffenbarger RS Jr, et al. The influence of physical activity on the incidence of site-specific cancers in college alumni. Adv Exp Med Biol 1992;322:7.

19. Uhlenbrock G, Oder U. Can endurance sports stimulate immune mechanisms against cancer and metastasis. Int J Sports Med 1991;12(suppl 1):S63.

20. Porock D, et al. An exercise intervention for advanced cancer patients experiencing fatigue: a pilot study. J Palliat Care 2000;16:30.

21. Segal R, et al. Structured Exercise improves Physical Functioning in Women with stages I and II Breast Cancer: Results of a Randomized Controlled Trial. J Clin Oncol 2001;19:657.

22. Winningham ML, et al. Effects of aerobic exercise on body weight and composition in patients with breast cancer on adjuvant chemotherapy. Oncol Nurs Forum 1989;16:683.

23. Brown JK. Gender, age, usual weight loss, and tobacco use as predictors of weight loss in patients with lung cancer. Oncol Nurs Forum 1993;20:466.

24. Dimeo F, et al. Aerobic exercise as therapy for cancer fatigue. Med Sci Sports Exerc 1998;30:475.

25. Sarna L. Functional status in women with cancer. Cancer Nurs 1994;17:87.

26. Segar ML, et al. The effect of aerobic exercise on self-esteem and depressive and anxiety symptoms among breast cancer survivors. Oncol Nurs Forum 1998;25:107.

27. Pedersen BK, et al. Exercise and the immune system – influence of nutrition and aging. J Sci Med Sport 1999;2:234

28. Jonsdottir IH, et al. Enhancement of natural immunity seen after voluntary exercise in rats. Role of central opioid receptors. Life Sci 2000;66:1231.

29. Mackinnon LT. Future directions in exercise and immunology: regulation and integration. Int J Sports Med 1998;19:S205.

30. Shephard RJ, Shek PN. Exercise, immunity, and susceptibility to infection. Phys Sportsmed 1999;27(6):47.

31. Bruunsgaard H, et al. In vivo cell-mediated immunity and vaccination response following prolonged, intense exercise. Med Sci Sports Exerc 1997;29:1176.

32. Davis JM, et al. Exercise, alveolar macrophage function, and susceptibility

to respiratory infection. J Appl Physiol 1997;83:1461.

33. Kajuura JS, et al. Immune responses to changes in training intensity and volume in runners. Med Sci Sports Exerc 1995;27:1111.

34. Koppel M, et al. Effects of elevated plasma noradrenaline concentration on the immune system in humans. Eur J Appl Physiol 1998;79:93.

35. Mackinnon LT, Jenkins DG. Decreased salivary immunoglobins after intense interval exercise before and after training. Med Sci Sports Exerc 1993;25:678.

36. Peters EM, et al. Vitamin C supplementation reduces the incidence of postrace symptoms of upper-respiratory-tract infection in ultra-marathon runners. Am J Clin Nutr 1993;57:170.

37. Shephard RJ, et al. The impact of exercise on the immune system: NK cells, interleukins 1 and 2, and related responses. Exerc Sport Sci Rev 1995;23:215.

38. Weinstock C, et al. Effect of exhaustive exercise stress on the cytokine response. Med Sci Sports Exerc 1997;29:345.

39. Fahlman M, et al. Effects of endurance training on selected parameters of immune function in elderly women. Gerontology 2000;46:97.

40. Scanga CB, et al. Effects of weight loss and exercise training on natural killer cell activity in obese women. Med Sci Sports Exerc 1998;30:1668.

41. Shephard RJ, Shek PN. Exercise, aging and immune function. Int J Sports Med 1995;16:1.

42. Neiman DC, et al. The acute immune response to exhaustive resistance exercise. Int J Sports Med 1995;16:322.

9

WHY EXERCISE?

To Prevent or Reverse Depression

Why Exercise? - To Prevent or Reverse Depression

Understanding Depression

Many people have described depression as a black curtain of despair coming down over their lives. Depressed people lose their ability to concentrate and have little to no energy most of the time. They become increasingly more irritable and often say to other people they are 'feeling low or down'. People who have been feeling 'down' for more than two weeks are generally described as "clinically depressed".

UK Statistics on Depression

An estimated 3.5 million people are suffering from major depression in the UK. But depression is not just diagnosed in adults now. These days, sadly, the incidence of depression among children and teenagers is also on the rise.

- **Major depression is the No.1 psychological disorder in the western world. It is growing in all age groups, in virtually every community, and the growth is mostly seen in the young, especially teens. At the current rate of increase, it will be the 2nd most disabling condition in the world by 2020, behind heart disease.** [1]

- **There is 10 times more major depression in people born after 1945 than in those born before. This clearly shows that the root cause of most depression is not a chemical imbalance. Human genes do not change that fast.** [1]

- People of all ages, backgrounds, lifestyles, and nationalities suffer from major depression, with a few exceptions. [1]

- As many as one person in three will experience an episode of depression at some point in their life. [2]

- The average age of first onset of major depression is 25-29. [1]

- Mixed anxiety & depression is the most common mental disorder in Britain, with almost 9 percent of people meeting the criteria for diagnosis. The Office for National Statistics Psychiatric Morbidity report (2001). [3]

- Between 8-12% of the population experience depression in any year. The Office for National Statistics Psychiatric Morbidity report

(2001). [3]

- Common antidepressant drugs could lead to osteoporosis, research from the US suggests. [4]
- The numbers of young people suffering from depression has risen in the last 10 years. Government statistics say depression now affects 1 in 10 young people. [5]

Symptoms of Depression

Forty-five to seventy-five percent of people who are diagnosed with mental depression experience physical symptoms such as stomach aches and indigestion; weight loss or weight gain; fatigue; aches and pain in the back, neck or shoulders; muscular stress and tension; sleeping too much or too little; and headaches. Being depressed can be emotionally suffocating. Symptoms such as prolonged sadness, loss of interest in life, an inability to make simple decisions, feeling overwhelmed and hopeless, are all emotional symptoms associated with depression.

What does Depression generally lead to?

Depression can lead to trouble concentrating or making life decisions and an inability to function well in everyday life. Work and interactions with family and friends can become increasingly more difficult. Prolonged depression can often lead to thoughts of suicide and the act of suicide itself.

Why Does It Happen?

Although the cause of depression is unknown, the condition is often triggered by too much mental stress from major life events. Major life events may include financial difficulties or work challenges, relationship difficulties, moving, divorce, or even the birth of a child.

Why Exercise?

Scientific Research on Depression & Exercise

According to the findings of a study conducted by Duke University Medical Center, **a brisk 30 minute walk or jog around a track three times a week may be just as effective in relieving the symptoms of major depression as anti-depressant medication**, the standard orthodox

medical treatment.

Researchers at Duke University studied a group of middle-aged and elderly individuals, but the results are likely to be congruent with individuals of any age. This is because, generally, elderly individuals can be the most difficult group on which to test an exercise hypothesis. Elderly people tend to have additional medical problems that can make regular exercise even more difficult. Therefore, the positive results in a test on elderly people seems to point to the likelihood of positive results among younger people as well.

Duke psychologist and lead researcher, James Blumenthal, looked closely at one of the results from the study that involved 156 elderly patients with major depressive disorder (MDD). He said that exercise may be just as effective as medication and may be a better alternative for some patients with MDD.

Blumenthal also suggested that the structured and supportive atmosphere of the study could have had a positive effect on improving the symptoms of the group. However, he believes that, whilst the camaraderie in the group may have contributed to the overall effect, the majority of the lasting benefit derived from the effects of the exercise programme.

How Exercise Works to Relieve Depression

Exercise may be effective in relieving depression because when patients choose to exercise, they are taking an active role in trying to 'get better.' This may be better than passively choosing to take a pill, and then sitting on the sofa watching TV and 'expecting' to get better. In the study, it became apparent that patients who exercised felt a greater sense of mastery over their condition. They, therefore, gained self-esteem and a sense of accomplishment because they were doing it for themselves.

In another study, Dr. Michael Craig Miller, Assistant Professor of Psychiatry at Harvard Medical School in Boston, Massachusetts said that vigorous exercise produces "helpful chemicals in the brain." These chemicals are known as endorphins, the chemicals responsible for the euphoric feelings associated with exercise. He also went on to say that improved self-esteem is also associated with regular physical activity, which can contribute to an enhanced sense of well-being. Therefore,

this combination of endorphins and improved self-esteem can be helpful in the relief of depression.

Increased participation in exercise is strongly associated with lowering levels of depression. [6] Regular low-to-moderate exercise can help to produce endorphins in the brain. When endorphin production improves, mood follows. [7] **It could be that the most important beneficial aspect of exercise is related to its ability to improve mood. This benefit is so critical because mental attitude is a critical factor in preventing illness and disease**. Regular exercise may actually be the most powerful antidepressant available. [8, 9, 10, 11, 12]

Many scientific studies to-date have clearly indicated that exercise is a profound antidepressant. They show that increased participation in exercise and physical activity decreases symptoms of anxiety and depression. They also show that people who participate in regular exercise feel better, are happier, and have higher self-esteem than those who do not. In fact, over 100 studies to date have identified the effectiveness of exercise in the treatment of depression.

In 1980, an analysis of sixty-four scientific studies that were concluded prior to 1980, confirmed that exercise relieves depression. [13]

Neurogenesis

Neurogenesis, or the birth of new neuronal cells, could be an important factor in the treatment of depression and also in everyday mood. It is now thought that neurogenesis can indeed continue into and throughout adult life, however research suggests that it is dependant on two key factors: physical exercise and human interaction.

A 1997 study conducted by Kemperman and Gage found that adult mice given enriched living conditions showed a sixty percent increase in new cell growth. Scientists are now studying how neurogenesis occurs naturally, and how it can be used to assist in various medical treatments. Neurogenesis is regulated by growth factors that can lead to the development of new cells. [14, 15, 16]

Neurotrophic Factors

Scientists have recently discovered a whole family of proteins called neurotrophic factors. The word "neurotrophic" is derived from the Greek

words "neuro" for nerve and "troph" for nourish. These proteins play a crucial role in the development and survival of nerve cells, or neurons. Neurotrophic factors are responsible for the growth and survival of neurons during development and also keep adult neurons alive and healthy throughout life.

The Division of Molecular Psychiatry at Yale School of Medicine studies demonstrated that stress and depression decrease neurotrophic factor expression and neurogenesis in the brain. In an article published on February 3rd 2006, they went on to say that neurotrophic factors and neurogenesis can decrease with age, but may <u>not</u> have to. The study says, "Exercise and an enriched environment increase neurotrophic support and neurogenesis, which could block the effects of stress and ageing."

The Department of Psychology, Division of Neuroscience and the Brain Research Centre at UBC Hospital, University of British Columbia, Vancouver, studies revealed that "an enriched environment and voluntary exercise massively increases neurogenesis in the adult hippocampus".

Many people today do not want to take anti-depressants. Reports conclude that more and more people are concerned about the side effects of drugs. These people are looking for more 'natural' ways of feeling better. In any case, the findings of these **studies confirm that exercise may be as effective as medication in the treatment of depression**. These findings may begin to pave the way for more research to be conducted, and could change the way depressed patients are treated in the future.

The Department of Medical-Surgical Nursing, University of Illinois, Chicago says, "the beneficial effects of both exercise and multi-sensory environmental stimulation have been well-documented."

An Enriched Environment

Dr. Marian C. Diamond is professor of anatomy at the Department of Integrative Biology, University of California. She is one of the world's foremost neuroanatomists. Dr. Diamond's work with rats has proved the importance of an enriched environment. This research is, without doubt, applicable to human learning. Diamond's work shows that 5 basic factors are important to keep a brain healthy well into old age.

Five basic factors for a healthy brain are:

- Human love

- Diet

- Exercise

- Challenge

- Newness

"The brain needs new challenges if it is to remain a healthy, functioning organ. At any age, trying more difficult tasks, especially those involving multisensory input (seeing, listening, feeling), is a good thing". Diamond further reports, "Because 'newness' is an important aspect of challenge, we changed the toys frequently in rat experiments; otherwise, the brain at first responds to the enriched conditions but decreases its growth activity when the newness wears off."

However, Diamond goes on to say that too much stimulation or newness causes stress, which has a negative impact on brain development. [17, 18, 19, 20, 21, 22]

In Summary:

- It is perfectly natural to become upset when life is challenging - everyone has their moments! Clinical depression, on the other hand, is a debilitating and often long lasting medical condition which is largely seen as a "modern" disease, affecting not only the sufferers themselves, but also those close to them.

- Whilst the causes of depression can be complex, the most common triggers are lifestyle related and can therefore be negated by developing more positive habits.

- There is absolutely no doubt that if you take regular physical exercise you will (in addition to the other health benefits) have a far more positive self image and find it easier to take life's knocks in your stride.

Chapter References

1. Depression Learning Path Major Depression Facts. Available from http://www.clinical-depression.co.uk/Depression_Information/facts.htm [cited 11 July 2007]

2. BBC July 2006 Depression. Available from http://www.bbc.co.uk/health/conditions/depression1.shtml [cited 11 July 2007]

3. Mental Health Foundation 2006 Statistics on Mental Health. Available from http://www.mentalhealth.org.uk/information/mental-health-overview/statistics/ [cited 11 July 2007]

4. Arthritis Research Campaign 10 July 2007 Antidepressants 'could add to osteoporosis risk'. Available from http://www.arc.org.uk/news/article/18206829 [cited 10th July 2007]

5. BBC Newsround 4 August 2004 Depression in children on the up. Available from http://news.bbc.co.uk/cbbcnews/hi/uk/newsid_3535000/3535680.stm [cited 11 July 2007]

6. U.S. Dept. of Health and Human Services, The Surgeon General's Report on Nutrition and Health (Rocklin, CA: Prima, 1988).

7. Daniel Carr et al., "Physical Conditioning Facilitates the Exercised-Induced-Secretion of Beta-Endorphin and Beta-Lipoprotein.

8. J.E. Martin and P.M. Dubbert, "Exercise Applications and Promotion in Behavioral Medicine," J Consult Clin Psychol 50 (1982): 1004-17.

9. C.H. Folkins and W.E. Sime, "Physical Fitness Training and Mental Health," Am Psychologist 36 (1981):375-88.

10. S.Weyerer and B. Kupfer, "Physical Exercise and Psychological Health," Sports Med 17 (1994): 108-16.

11. A. Byrne and D.G. Byrne, "The Effect of Exercise on Depression, Anxiety, and Other Mood States: A Review," J Psychosom Res 37 (1993): 565-74.

12. R.C. Casper. "Exercise and Mood," World Rev Nutr Diet 71 (1993):115-43.

13. C.H. Folkins and W.E. Sime, Physical Fitness Training and Mental Health," Am Psychologist 36 (1981): 375-88.

14. Gage, Fred. (2003). Brain, Repair Yourself. Scientific American, 289(3), 87-95.

15. Kempermann and Gage (2003). New Nerve Cells for the Adult Brain. (2003) Retrieved 11, 03, 2003 From: http://www.dsrf.co.uk/Reading_material/New_braincells/newbrain2.htm.

16. Eriksson et al. (1998). Neurogenesis in the adult human hippocampus. Nature America Inc. Retrieved 11, 03, 2003 from: http://medicine.nature.com

17. Bennett E L, Rosenzweig M R, Diamond M C 1974 "Effects of successive environments on brain measures." Physio. and Behavior 12:621-631

18. Carughi A, Carpenter K J, Diamond M C 1990 "The Developing Cerebral

Cortex: nutritional and environmental influences." Malnutrition and the Infant Brain. Wiley-Liss p.127-139

19. Diamond M C, Krech D, Rosenzweig M R 1964 "The effects of an Enriched Environment on the Rat Cerebral Cortex." J. Comp. Neurol. 123:111-119

20. Diamond M C, Connor J R, Orenberg E K, Bissell M, Yost M, Krueger A 1980 "Environmental Influences on Serotonin and Cyclic Nucleotides in Rat Cerebral Cortex." Science 210:652-654

21. Diamond M C, Greer E R, York A, Lewis D, Barton T, Lin J 1987 "Rat Cortical Morphology Following Crowded-Enriched Living Conditions." Exp. Neurol. 96:241-247

22. Diamond M C, 1988 Enriching Heredity, The Free Press, New York

WHY EXERCISE?

To Prevent or Reverse Diabetes

Why Exercise? - To Prevent or Reverse Diabetes

Understanding Diabetes

Diabetes mellitus can be broken down into two subgroups: insulin-dependant diabetes (type 1) and non insulin-dependant diabetes (type 2).

Type 1 diabetes, also known as juvenile-onset diabetes, usually occurs in younger people. This form of diabetes results from an autoimmune response. [1]

Type 2 diabetes tends to affect people over age 40. However, many overweight children are now also being affected, some as young as 10 years of age. [2]

Diabetes results from the body's inability to respond properly to insulin. [3] In diabetes, individuals have high blood sugar levels. The reason for this is that the sugar in the blood is not getting into the cells where it is needed.

Once inside the cell, the sugar needs to be transported inside the mitochondria, which is like the engine of the cell. For diabetics, this process does not happen as efficiently. In healthy individuals, once the sugar gets inside the mitochondria it meets and mixes with oxygen and combustion occurs. Heat occurs as a result of the combustion and this produces power.

This is how electricity is made in the human body and how the human body produces energy. However, when this process does not happen efficiently, electricity is not generated and therefore energy is not produced efficiently.

UK Statistics on Diabetes

Diabetes is a globally serious problem in the modern world, (in the USA, for example, there are an estimated 16 million people already diagnosed with diabetes with another estimated 8 - 16 million people suffering but as yet undiagnosed).

Studies suggest that the disease has tripled in children in the last 3 to 5 years. Type 2 diabetes accounts for over 95% of all diabetes cases in the world. [4] Diabetes, obesity and hypertension (high blood pressure) are inter-related and **the combination of high blood pressure and being overweight increases the chances of developing diabetes ten-fold**.

- Overall, 4% of men and 3% of women in England have diagnosed diabetes. Prevalence increases with age. [4]

- Prevalence is also increasing. **Diabetes has more than doubled in men and increased by 80% in women since 1991**. [4]

- Extrapolations suggest around 7% of men and 5% of women will have diabetes by 2010. [4]

- **There are more than 2 million people known to have diabetes in the UK and it's estimated that well over a million people have the condition without being aware of it**. [5]

- Around 15% of heart attacks in Western Europe are due to diagnosed diabetes. [4]

- More than twice the number of Black Caribbean and Indian men have diabetes than the general population. 2.5 times the number of Black Caribbean and Pakistani women have diabetes than the general population. The prevalence in Black African and Irish women is substantially lower. [4]

Symptoms of Diabetes

Type 1 diabetes usually develops very quickly, over a few weeks, so symptoms appear very quickly. Generally, type 2 diabetes develops over a period of years, so many people may not notice any signs of the developing illness. Others may pass off their symptoms as the result of overwork or age.

The main symptoms of diabetes are: increased thirst, extreme tiredness, going to the toilet all the time (especially at night), unexplained weight loss, genital itching or regular episodes of thrush, blurred vision and slow healing of cuts and wounds.

What does Diabetes generally lead to?

Diabetes is the leading cause of blindness, kidney failure and limb amputations. Research indicates diabetes is a major risk factor for cardiovascular disease, and therefore cancer and early death. [6]

Why Does it Happen?

Diabetes is linked to poor diet, lack of physical activity, alcohol, smoking and obesity. Fortunately, diabetes experts believe that lifestyle changes can significantly reduce the risk of developing diabetes. Those who have developed type 2 diabetes can also benefit from lifestyle changes, especially those related to diet and exercise and other changes that will promote the maintenance of a healthy body weight.

Why Exercise?

Scientific Research on Diabetes & Exercise

Data from cross-sectional research provides strong evidence that regular exercise reduces type 2 diabetes, with or without body composition changes. [7, 8, 9, 10] Obese, sedentary and hypertensive individuals have the greatest risk of developing diabetes, however, in studies it is also these individuals who receive the greatest benefits from regular exercise. [2, 11] [12, 13] Studies confirm that middle-aged men who exercise reduce blood pressure and improve glucose and fat metabolism, which contributes to reduced risk of diabetes and cardiovascular disease. [14]

One 6-year clinical trial evaluated the effects of dietary and exercise lifestyle interventions on individuals with type 2 diabetes. The results were conclusive: diet, exercise and combined diet-exercise interventions significantly decreased type 2 diabetes. [15]

A study of the Pima tribe of Adult Native American Indians found they have 10 to 15 times more type 2 diabetes than the general U.S. population! The data was analysed against their participation in physical activity. It concluded that, regardless of body mass, physical activity is essential to avoid type 2 diabetes. [16, 17]

Scientific studies show that improved insulin sensitivity is one of the most important benefits of regular physical activity. [18] Exercise also increases the liver's insulin sensitivity. [19] Endurance and resistance training combined have improved the health of insulin-resistant individuals more than endurance training alone. [20] The reason for this increased benefit seems to be the fact that these combined exercise programmes activate a greater volume of overall body muscle mass. [21]

Dr. William Knowler, of the National Institute of Diabetes and Digestive Kidney Diseases, conducted a study on diabetes. Knowler's study, published in The New England Journal, found that lifestyle changes decreased the risk factor for the development of diabetes by 58 percent. The study contrasted this finding with the performance of treatment with metaformin (Glucophage or Glucovance by Bristol-Myers Squibb), which only reduced the risk by 31 percent.

The study also found that lifestyle changes did not have to be drastic to make a difference. Just 2.5 hours of exercise a week combined with healthier eating habits was enough to produce significant benefits.

Dr. Ming Wei and associates from The Cooper Institute in Dallas, Texas studied men with type 2 diabetes. Those who were active and physically fit had a lower overall risk of dying than diabetic men who led sedentary lifestyles. Wei said, "Doctors should encourage patients with type 2 diabetes to participate in regular aerobic exercise."

Dr. Charles Clark Jr. from Richard Roudebush Veterans Affairs Medical Center in Indianapolis reviewed the results of 1,263 men with type 2 diabetes.

Dr. Clark reported that unfit individuals are:

- More likely to die from diabetes
- Twice as likely to die from heart disease
- 2.4 times more likely to die from cancer
- 5 times more likely to die from digestive disease

Based on these results, he concluded in an editorial, "The data supporting the health benefits of physical activity are overwhelming."

The results from another study, conducted by The University of Queensland found that Tai Chi had a beneficial effect on indicators of glucose metabolism. The Queensland study also found that Tai Chi could be used as a preventive measure for type 2 diabetes. The team of researchers found that the spiral movements of Tai Chi might possibly stimulate muscles more effectively than conventional exercises. These movements might lead to greater uptake and utilisation of glucose.

One serious symptom of diabetes, the slow healing of cuts and wounds, may also improve with exercise. The body's ability to heal from wounds

lessens as we age, but a study published in the Journal of Gerontology: Medical Sciences revealed **regular exercise can speed up the wound-healing process by as much as 25 percent**. Charles Emery, Professor of Psychology was the lead author of the Ohio State University study.

A recent study, published in 2006, showed that obese and overweight individuals suffering from type 2 diabetes experienced significant health improvements after only three weeks of moderate exercise and diet. An interesting note about these participants is that if they remained obese or overweight, they still experienced positive results.

This study, involving 31 men, was lead by Christian Roberts of the University of California, Los Angeles. Roberts showed that, **contrary to generally accepted medical research and belief, type 2 diabetes can be reversed solely through lifestyle changes**. The lifestyle changes paramount in the study were simply moderate exercise and healthier eating habits. The men ate a more balanced, healthier diet. They also exercised on a treadmill (with level and graded walking) for 45-60 minutes a day.

Angiogenesis

Angiogenesis refers to the process by which new blood vessels are formed within the body. When tissues need more oxygen, for example, they release molecules that encourage blood vessels to grow.

Blood in the body is pumped through arteries and smaller vessels to every corner of the body. There should be a capillary network in between arteries and blood vessels. Capillaries are tiny blood vessels that interlink to form networks. Capillary density is essential for healthy blood supply to every part of the body.

If an individual has good capillary density, they should experience no problems with blood circulation and supply. However, a lack of capillary density can create a lack of oxygen supply and this can decrease the provision of nutrients to the cells near areas of low capillary density.

The Department of Physiology & Pharmacology, Karolinska Institute, Stockholm, Sweden, says, "**Angiogenesis is a common adaptive response to exercise training in skeletal muscle**. Recent studies have shown that angiogenesis occurs in response to increased muscle activity in skeletal

muscle."

Diabetics generally lose capillary density as the high levels of sugar in the blood damage the capillaries. When an individual lacks capillary density, adverse effects of poor blood circulation crop up throughout the body. Capillaries shrink with excess amounts of sugar, so blood cannot flow easily or efficiently.

It has long been recognized that individuals who do <u>not</u> exercise have a lower number of mitochondria in their cells. In fact, individuals with long-term sedentary lifestyles usually have very low mitochondria levels. **A decline in mitochondria increases the risk of developing diabetes by ten times**. Therefore, to keep mitochondria levels high, individuals should perform aerobic and resistance training exercises regularly.

Stretching is another component of training that combats diabetes. Exercise Physiologists have found that flexibility is critically important, because our health depends upon our circulation. No matter how well you eat, if you do not have good circulation, the delivery of oxygen and nutrients to your cells may be poor.

Capillaries extend to the parts of the body that are regularly used (regularly sending signals requesting oxygen and nourishment). If a part of the body is not used, capillaries shrink and diminish in number. This causes cells to perform poorly and even atrophy or die. For optimal blood circulation and health, capillary density throughout the entire body is critically important.

To maintain capillary density within every part of the body, all parts of the body must be used regularly. If an individual stretches regularly and is therefore flexible, there should an abundance of capillary density throughout the body. If an individual is not flexible there may <u>not</u> be an abundance of oxygen and nutrient supply to some of the tissues throughout the body. Tight, unused areas of the body, where flexibility is not optimal due to a lack of exercise/stretching/flexibility may also lack capillary density and therefore circulation (an abundant supply of oxygen and nutrients).

In Summary:

- As with many other diseases, diabetes is fast becoming a global epidemic, the health consequences of which are profound and far-reaching. This is, once again, predominantly due to the poor lifestyle choices of modern man – in particular, inappropriate diet and lack of physical activity.

- However, there is clear, irrefutable evidence that regular exercise is a powerful defence against the disease and can even, in some cases, materially reverse existing conditions. So, it's never too soon – or too late - to start a defined exercise programme for optimum health.

Chapter References

1. Yoon J-W, et al. Control of autoimmune diabetes in NOD mice by GAD expression or suppression in cells. Science 1999;284:1183.

2. Gower BA, et al. Fat distribution and insulin in prepubertal African American and white children. Am J Clin Nutr 1998;67:821.

3. Simoneau J-A, et al. Altered glycolytic and oxidative capacities of skeletal muscle contribute to insulin resistance in NIDDM. J Appl Physiol 1997;83:166.

4. Allender, S., Peto, V., Scarborough, P., Boxer, A., Rayner, M. (2006) Coronary Heart Disease Statistics. British Heart Foundation, London.

5. BBC Diabetes. Available from http://www.bbc.co.uk/health/conditions/diabetes/ [cited 11 July 2007]

6. Grundy SM, et al. Diabetes and cardiovascular disease: a statement for health professionals from the American Heart Association. Circulation 1999;100:1134.

7. American College of Sports Medicine. Position Stand. Exercise and type 2 diabetes. Med Sci Sports Exerc 32:1345;2000.

8. Vukovich MD, et al. Changes in insulin action and GLUT-4 with 6 days of inactivity in endurance runners. J Appl Physiol 1996;80:240.

9. Wannamethee, S.G., et al. Physical activity, metabolic factors, and the incidence of coronary heart disease and type 2 diabetes. Arch Intern Med 160:2108, 2000.

10. White RD, Sherman C. Exercise in diabetes management: maximizing benefits, controlling risks. Phys Sportsmed 1999;27(4):63.

11. ADA/ACSM. Diabetes mellitus and exercise joint position paper. Med Sci Sports Exerc 1997;29:I.

12. Kriska AM, et al. The potential role of physical activity in the prevention of non-insulin-dependant diabetes mellitus: the epidemiological evidence. Exerc

Sport Sci Rev 1994;22:21.

13. Pan X, et al. Effects of diet and exercise in preventing NIDDM in people with impaired glucose tolerance: the DaQuing and Diabetes Study. Diabetes Care. 1997;20:537.

14. Dengel DR, et al. Improvements in blood pressure, glucose metabolism, and lipoprotein lipids after aerobic exercise plus weight loss in obese, hypertensive middle-aged men. Metabolism 1998;47:1075.

15. Xiao-ren P, et al. Effects of diet and exercise in preventing NIDDM in people with impaired glucose tolerance. Diabetes Care. 1997;20:537.

16. Kriska Am, et al. The association of physical activity with obesity, fat distribution and glucose intolerance in Pima Indians. Diabetologia 1993;36:863.

17. Manson JD, et al. A prospective study of exercise and incidence of diabetes among US male physicians. JAMA 1992;268:63.

18. Mayer-Davis EJ, et al. Intensity and amount of physical activity in relation to insulin sensitivity. JAMA 1998;279:669.

19. Devlin JT, et al. Enhanced peripheral and splanchnic insulin sensitivity in NIDDM men after a single bout of exercise. Diabetes 1987;36:434.

20. Wallace MB, et al. Effects of cross-training on markers of insulin resistance/hyperinsulinemia. Med Sci Sports Exerc 1997;29:1170.

21. Arciero PJ, et al. Effects of short-term inactivity on glucose tolerance, energy expenditure, and blood flow in trained subjects. J Appl Physiol 1998;84:1365.

WHY
EXERCISE?
To Prevent or
Reverse Arthritis

Why Exercise? - To Prevent or Reverse Arthritis

Understanding Arthritis

The term arthritis covers a number of degenerative and inflammatory conditions that cause pain, inflammation and stiffness in joints. In the modern world, arthritis is at an all-time high. Many people believe this increase may be due to poor diet, sedentary lifestyles, and injuries from competitive sports.

Joints, where bones meet, allow our bodies to move, to be flexible. The ends of bones are covered by a lubricated tissue we call cartilage. During movement, the lubricated cartilage tissue prevents the friction of bone grinding against bone. It serves, in essence, as a cushion or pad between bones. This cushion assures that the bones do not wear out. Fibrous ligaments that surround joints provide strength, stabilise and support joints, and prevent excessive movement.

Unlike other body tissues, there is no blood supply to cartilage (there is no nerve supply either). Cartilage receives its necessary nutrients to stay in good condition from bodily fluids, which move around the joint when the joint is moved through its full range of motion.

To promote joint health, proper joint movement is essential. This movement transports nutrients to the cartilage effectively. Clinical studies have shown that nonstcroidal anli-inflammatory drugs (NSAIDs) such as Ibubrofen, Nurpin, etc. suppress the symptoms but accelerate the progression of osteoarthritis. NSAIDs accelerate cartilage destruction, osteoarthritis progression and joint deterioration. [1, 2, 3, 4]

Nutrition is important. If you are not eating the right oils, then your cartilage can become dry. Dry cartilage can start to deteriorate, and this can quickly lead to the onset of degenerative arthritis.

Types of Arthritis

Osteoarthritis

Osteoarthritis is the most common form of arthritis. It is estimated that in the UK alone, 80 percent of people over the age of 50 have osteoarthritis. It is a progressive, degenerative, painful 'wear and tear' disease.

In osteoarthritis, the protective cartilage found at the end of bones wears away. With less cartilage, the bone ends around the joint thicken through friction and bony growths or osteophytes (large bone spurs) may form. This deformation is what often makes the joint appear larger or swollen.

With the formation of osteophytes, the synovial fluid in the joint becomes less able to lubricate the joint properly. As a result, the whole joint area then becomes inflamed and the joint's ability to work properly is decreased. Decreased work ability restricts joint movement; increasing stiffness and tenderness and creates pain.

It is known that the primary cause of osteoarthritis is repeated joint damage from strenuous activity or sports competitions. Wear quickly occurs in joints that are over-exercised with movements that are executed for the purpose of winning, and are thus impulsive, fast, rigorous and strenuous. In studies, osteoarthritis is common in former athletes, ballet dancers, and gymnasts. Damaging a joint early in life may lead to the development of osteoarthritis later on.

Obesity places extra stress on joints and therefore increases a person's risk of developing a joint disorder and osteoarthritis. [5, 6] At the same time, building too much extra muscular bulk (body-building), can cause the extra muscle tissue to alter the natural alignment of joints, encouraging joints to deteriorate.

Rheumatoid Arthritis

Rheumatoid Arthritis is an autoimmune disorder. When an individual is healthy, the immune system can distinguish between healthy body tissues and foreign unhealthy organisms, such as bacteria and viruses. With an autoimmune disorder, the immune system loses its ability to distinguish between unhealthy and healthy cells, and by mistake attacks its body's own tissues.

Ankylosing Spondylitis

Another form of arthritis is Spondylitis, a persistent disease that usually affects the spine and pelvis. The stiffening and inflammation of joints from this disease is four times more common in men than in women. If Ankylosing Spondylitis is left untreated, the spine can distort and new bone actually grows between the vertebrae, which can eventually fuse

together.

UK Statistics on Arthritis

Arthritis is the second most common cause of time off work in the UK.

- There are over 200 kinds of rheumatic diseases (the word "rheumatic" means aches and pains in joints, bones and muscles). Two of the most common forms of arthritis are osteoarthritis and rheumatoid arthritis. [7]

- Over nine million people in the UK have arthritis. [7]

- Arthritis is not just a disease of older people – it can affect people of all ages, including children. It is not clear what causes arthritis and there is no cure at present. However, there is plenty you can do to manage your condition and lead a full and active life. [7]

- There are 12,000 children in the UK with arthritis and approximately 27,000 people living with arthritis are under the age of 25 (Arthritis Research Campaign 2002). Around half of those with musculoskeletal conditions are under the age of 65, based on prevalence rates by age. (Office for National Statistics, 2002). [8]

- Common antidepressant drugs could lead to osteoporosis, research from the US suggests. [9]

The human cost of arthritis and related conditions. (1)

- More than 7 million adults in the UK (15% of the population) have long-term health problems due to arthritis and related conditions. [10]

- Almost 9 million people in the UK (19% of the population) visited their GP in the past year with arthritis and related conditions. [10]

- More than 2 million people visited their GP in the past year because of osteoarthritis. The number of people with osteoarthritis has risen over the past 10 years as the population ages, and more people are now seeking their GP's help. [10]

- At least 4.4 million people in the UK have X-ray evidence of moderate to severe osteoarthritis in their hands; 550,000 have moderate to severe osteoarthritis in their knees; and 210,000 have moderate to severe osteoarthritis of the hips. [10]

- **Obesity is a major risk factor for osteoarthritis of the knee. The UK currently has the eighth highest obesity rate in the world - and this is**

rising. [10]

- Around 387,000 people in the UK have rheumatoid arthritis - roughly 0.8% of the adult population. There are around 12,000 new cases a year. [10]

- Around 12,000 children have juvenile idiopathic arthritis in the UK. [10]

- Each year 200,000 people visit their GP with ankylosing spondylitis. (2) [10]

- Around 2.6 million people in the UK visited their GP with back pain in the past year. [10]

- Almost nine-tenths of people with arthritis or joint pain (87%) are not under the care of a rheumatologist or orthopaedic surgeon. [10]

- Two-thirds of people with arthritis (66%) are satisfied with the level of care and treatment they receive from their GP. [10]

- **Arthritis and related conditions are the second most common cause of days off work in both men and women**. [10]

- More than 44,000 hip replacements and more than 35,000 knee replacements were performed in the UK in 2000. [10]

- 50% of people with arthritis say the worst aspect is pain. This rises to 55% of people with osteoarthritis. [10]

The cost to the nation of arthritis and related conditions:

- **206 million working days were lost in the UK in 1999-2000 due to arthritis alone**. [10]

- £2.4 billion was paid in incapacity benefit in 2001. [10]

- £98 million was paid to people claiming severe disablement allowance in 2001. [10]

- Cost of community and social services was £389 million and £1.3 billion respectively in 2001. [10]

- Cost of GP consultations was £307 million in 2000. [10]

- Cost of drugs prescribed was £341 million in 2000. [10]

- Cost of hip and knee replacements was £405 million in 2000. [10]

- **Total arthritis-related costs totalled in excess of £5.5 billion in 2000**. [10]

(1) The term 'musculoskeletal conditions' includes all conditions that

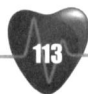

affect the bones, joints, and ligaments such as arthritis of all kinds, connective tissue diseases, back pain, osteoporosis, soft tissue rheumatism and regional and widespread pain. For the purpose of this book, arthritis and related conditions is used as an umbrella term to cover all these conditions. [10]

(2) There are no prevalence studies of ankylosing spondylitis in the UK. [10]

Symptoms of Arthritis

Pain tells you there is something wrong with your body. Generally, arthritis causes pain in joints. Pain from arthritis can affect different parts of the body and therefore prevent mobility. For example, someone who has arthritis of the elbow may experience swelling, pain and a decrease in motion available in the affected elbow joint.

Common symptoms of arthritis are: stiffness in and around joints early in the morning; swelling in joints; difficulty moving a joint through a full range of motion and constant or recurring tenderness or pain in joints.

What does Osteoarthritis generally lead to?

Arthritis is usually chronic, meaning it can occur over a long period of time. Pain in joints over time can dramatically affect a person's life. The chronic pain of arthritis often leads to chronic fatigue, loss of mobility, hospitalisation, joint replacements and early death.

Why Does it Happen?

Without proper exercise, diet and lifestyle habits, joints can become damaged, injured and worn. This causes them to lose their ability to function properly. Joints adapt to the daily activities and movements we perform.

Why Exercise?

Scientific Research on Arthritis & Exercise

If we do not use our joints through their full range of motion regularly, they will lose their full mobility, and the onset of a form of arthritis will occur. Nutrients are supplied to the cartilage by the continual movement of the joint. Therefore, without exercise, joints become less supple and lose

their full mobility. They naturally decline in health as you age, unless you exercise.

To cope with arthritis, the British Medical Journal (BMJ) recommends gentle, regular exercise to improve mobility and relieve stiffness. It also suggests that physical activity will strengthen the muscles that support joints. Muscles need to be exercised without straining joints, which almost completely rules out competitive sports for prevention and relief of arthritis.

In studies conducted to determine which kinds of exercises may be able to halt or even reverse osteoarthritis, results showed that the best types of exercises are those that increase circulation to joints and strengthen surrounding muscles without placing excessive strain on joints. [11] Walking programmes improve joint function in the knee and reduce pain. [12] Physical activities that overly strain joints – such as competitive sports – should be avoided to minimise arthritis in later life.

In Summary:

- **Everybody knows someone who suffers from some form of musculoskeletal disease, typically either osteoarthritis or rheumatoid arthritis. Traditionally thought of as a disease of the elderly, these complaints are now increasingly afflicting the young as well. Once again, the root causes are poor nutrition and lack of exercise.**

- **The good news is that by developing a lifetime habit of good physical activity, thus strengthening one's muscles, joints and ligaments and improving circulation, we can all reduce the likelihood of suffering from arthritis in later life. Moreover, it is clear that moderate physical activity can greatly alleviate the symptoms of existing arthritic conditions.**

Chapter References

1. P.M. Brooks, S.R Potter, and W.W. Buchanan, "NSAID and Osteoarthritis – Help or Hindrance," J Rheumatol 9 (1982): 3-5.

2. N.M. Newman and R.S.M. Ling, "Acetabular Bone Destruction Related to Non-Steriodal Anti-Inflammatory Drugs," Lancet 2 (1985): 11-13.

3. L. Solomon, "Drug Induced Arthropathy and Necrosis of the Femoral Head,"

J Bone Joint Surg 55B (1973): 246-51.

4. H. Ronningen and N. Langeland, "Indomethacin Treatment in Osteoarthritis of the Hip Joint," Acta Orthop Scand 50 (1979): 169-74.

5. A.J. Hartz, M.E. Fischer, G. Bril et al., "The Association of Obesity with Joint Pain and Osteoarthritis in the Hanes Data," J Chron Dis 39 (1986): 311-9.

6. D.T. Felson et al., "Weight Loss Reduces the Risk for Symptomatic Knee Osteoarthritis in Women," Ann Intern Med 116 (1992): 535-9.

7. Arthritis care. Available from http://www.arthritiscare.org.uk/AboutArthritis [cited 10th July 2007]

8. Back Care Key facts about Musculoskeletal Conditions. Available from http://www.backpain.org/pages/a_pages/arma-mscs.php [cited 10 July 2007]

9. Arthritis Research Campaign 10 July 2007 Antidepressants 'could add to osteoporosis risk'. Available from http://www.arc.org.uk/news/article/18206829 [cited 10th July 2007]

10. Arthritis Research Campaign May 2002 Arthritis Statistics. Available from http://www.arc.org.uk/arthinfo/astats.asp [cited 10 July 2007]

11. N.M. Fisher, D.R. Pendergast, and G.E. Gresham, "Muscle Rehabilitation: its Effects on Muscular and Functional Performance of Patients with Knee Osteoporosis," Arch Phys Med Rehabil 72 (1991): 367-74.

12. P.A. Kovar et al. "Supervised Fitness Walking in Patients with Osteoarthritis of the Knee: A randomized controlled trial," Ann Intern Med 116 (1992): 529-34.

WHY EXERCISE?

To Prevent or Reverse Osteoporosis

Why Exercise? - To Prevent or Reverse Osteoporosis

Understanding Osteoporosis

As we age, bones become increasingly more brittle and porous. Osteoporosis literally means "porous bones" and osteoporosis naturally develops over time. As we grow older, bones lose their mineral mass (bone mineral content) and calcium concentration (bone mineral density).

Bone exists in a continual state of flux. Bones are constantly remodeling, or going through a bone-destruction-and-building cycle. Remodeling breaks down old bone and replaces it with new bone. Bone-destroying cells (osteoclasts) cause the breakdown of bone, and bone-forming osteoblast cells induce new bone creation (synthesis).

Osteoporosis occurs when too much old bone is broken down and not enough new bone is rebuilt. **It is important to understand that just a 5% loss in bone mass increases the risk of a stress fracture by nearly 40%.** [1]

UK Statistics on Osteoporosis

Osteoporosis affects an estimated 75 million people in Europe, USA and Japan. Globally, osteoporosis is nearing epidemic proportions.

- About three million people in the UK have the condition, which is more common in women than men. [2]

- After the menopause, bone loss speeds up, making osteoporosis more likely. In women the risk is increased if they have an early menopause, have their ovaries removed before the menopause, or miss periods for six months or more as a result of excessive exercising or dieting. [2]

- For men low levels of testosterone increase the risk. [2]

- For men and women, long-term use of corticosteroid medication, maternal osteoporosis, smoking, heavy drinking, sedentary lifestyle, low body weight and medical conditions that affect absorption, such as coeliac disease, all increase the risk. [2]

In a report released in 2004, Stanford University School of Medicine expressed the concern that **millions of osteoporosis sufferers are undiagnosed and untreated**. The report also explained that **most sufferers learn of their disease only after they suffer a fracture**. Randall Stafford, MD, PhD, Assistant Professor of Medicine in the Stanford Prevention Research Centre, led a study ascertaining that fewer than half of the people with osteoporosis have been diagnosed or recognised as having this disease.

Symptoms of Osteoporosis

There are no real symptoms of osteoporosis. You cannot feel your bones lose mass and become weak. In fact, individuals can lose bone mass over many years and not know about it. For this reason, osteoporosis is often referred to as the 'silent disease.' Unfortunately, most people are not aware they are suffering bone loss until they fracture their spine or hip in a fall.

What does Osteoporosis generally lead to?

Every year in the UK, many individuals suffer hip and spine fractures due to osteoporosis. These fractures lead to hospitalisation and incapacitation, and even early death.

Why Does it Happen?

A lack of exercise stimulation (sedentary lifestyles) that can enhance bone strength is thought to be a primary cause of osteoporosis. However, poor nutrition, particularly insufficient intake of calcium, is another cause.

Why Exercise?

Scientific Research on Osteoporosis & Exercise

Many studies show that bone mass naturally decreases with age, but this process can be slowed with good nutrition and by implementing an exercise programme that incorporates 'high-impact' exercises.

More importantly, it's increasingly evident that with regard to avoiding osteoporosis – much more so than with any other chronic disease –

activities during childhood can benefit the person's future. A specific high-impact exercise programme implemented at an early age can put extra bone mass 'in the bank.' Children who have built up extra bone mass will obviously be far less likely to suffer from osteoporosis in the future.

Older women have an increased susceptibility to osteoporosis which coincides with menopause. [3] Proper nutrition, with particular attention to calcium intake and regular exercise can help women to maintain bone health later in life. [4, 5] However, it is the early teen years that serve as the primary years for maximising bone mass. [6, 7]

Adequate calcium intake is not the only important lifelong defence against bone loss. [8, 9, 10, 11] Regular exercise also slows the rate of skeletal ageing. **Individuals who exercise regularly have significantly greater bone mass than sedentary individuals**. [12, 13, 14, 15, 16, 17, 18, 19] It has been confirmed that regular exercise, early in life, often pays off into the seventh and eighth decades of life. [20] In addition, **the accelerated bone loss that usually accompanies weight reduction in postmenopausal women can be reversed with regular exercise**. [21]

Exercise training, specifically exercise that generates significant intermittent force against the body's long bones (walking, running and rope skipping) improve bone mass in adults. [22, 23, 24, 25, 26] However, individuals who performed high-impact exercise (such as volleyball, basketball and gymnastics) had the greatest bone mass. [27] In studies, the exercise effects are site-specific to the working muscles and the bones to which they are attached. [28]

Charles H. Turner is a professor in the Department of Orthopaedic Surgery and Director of Orthopaedic Research at Indiana University of Medicine, Indianapolis. According to his research, "Exercise that puts the 'best' kind of load to strengthen bones (especially during childhood or adolescence) involves impact or high rates of load such as jumping, as opposed to biking."

Turner goes on to state that the strengthening of bones through exercise is very efficient because the cellular mechanosensors within bone direct osteogenesis (new bone growth). This direction "tells" the body where new bone is needed most in order to improve bone strength and, hence, bone mass.

Impact-Loading Exercise

A study at Oregon State University (OSU) proved how children as young as 7 years old can significantly increase bone mass through regular exercise. But the critical component of the weekly exercise programme was that it contained "impact loading" exercises. Specifically, exercises that boost bone density in targeted areas – especially the hips.

In the research group, young volunteers jumped off two-foot boxes 100 times, three times a week for seven months. At the end of the study, the young volunteers who were jumping off the boxes had 5 percent more bone mass than individuals who were using their exercise time to stretch, or were performing non-impact exercise.

The principal investigator in this study was Director of the Bone Research Laboratory at OSU, Christine Snow. Snow said, "A five percent increase may not sound like a lot, but it translates into a 30 percent decrease in the risk of a hip fracture in adulthood."

The conclusions drawn from this research study (done in 1998) are very important. At that time, there had only been one other published study done in the world detailing how children could increase their bone mass. Unfortunately, that other study lacked clarity.

The unclear study, conducted in Australia, studied the bone mass of children who performed weight-lifting and jumping exercises for 50 minutes at a time, three times a week, for 10 months. The results showed similar gains of 5 to 8 percent in bone mass. However, it was unclear whether the jumping or the weight-lifting caused the increase in mass.

More recent research into bone mass points to the same conclusion – the best way to increase bone mass is through high-impact exercise. But the whole body needs to be strengthened, not just the hips. Jumping obviously will strengthen the hip area, but it is not a holistic approach. The exercise of jumping ignores the entire upper body (arms and shoulder joints), which will not benefit directly from the impact.

Improving Existing Bone Mass

Researchers at Johns Hopkins determined a moderate programme of physical exercise maintains bone mass, and in some cases, may offer modest improvements. The researchers found that exercise may

demonstrate significant increases in bone mass. Their study was the first to evaluate the effects of exercise, independent of other factors, primarily diet.

The study's lead investigator was Exercise Physiologist, Kerry Stewart, Ed.D. Kerry is Professor of Medicine and Director of Clinical Exercise Physiology and Heart Health Programmes at The Johns Hopkins University School of Medicine. Stewart assessed participants of an exercise programme which spanned a six-month period. At the end of this time, bone scans, using an X-ray machine called DXZ, were used to assess bone mineral density.

The Georgia Prevention Institute, Medical College of Georgia said in a report that physical activity, aerobic fitness, and strength have all been correlated with bone density. Young people who use a specific part of their body in vigorous exercise exhibit enhanced bone density in that part of the body, but not necessarily in other regions.

Most studies using specific bone-loading exercises have shown substantial increases in bone density at the specific sites loaded. However, extremely high volumes of exercise may overwhelm a person's adaptive capacity, leading to stress fractures. For example, young women athletes who suffer from menstrual dysfunction exhibit reduced bone density and musculoskeletal disorders.

NASA confirms that cosmonauts and astronauts who spend many months on the Space Station, Mir, lose (on average) 1 to 2 percent of bone mass each month. This weakening of the bones, often referred to as 'space bones' is a potentially serious side-effect of extended spaceflight. Dr. Jay Shapiro, team leader for bone studies at the National Space Biomedical Research Institute says, "The magnitude of this effect has led NASA to consider bone loss an inherent risk of extended space flights."

Researchers suspect that the root cause of bone loss in space is weightlessness. Scientists think reduced stress on bones may be responsible for the progressive bone loss seen in long-term residents of space. Lack of stress on bones among sedentary people on Earth, such as those confined to beds due to illness or old age, also contributes to bone loss. In space, bones are subject to prolonged exposure to zero-G. This has a negative impact on human bones, causing them to weaken.

Judith Cranford, The National Osteoporosis Foundation's (NOF) Executive Director says, "Parents should pay special attention to their children's bone health." She went on to say that children need to get enough weight-bearing exercise to promote bone health.

In Summary:

- Osteoporosis – the process by which our bones lose density and become more brittle – is sadly an inevitable by-product of ageing – to an extent.

- Just as poor nutritional habits and lack of exercise can accelerate this degeneration, better lifestyle choices can greatly reduce our chances of seeing our abilities and quality of life affected by the condition.

- In particular, an appropriate exercise routine which emphasises high impact activity and improves circulation may be the best defence of all.

Chapter References

1. Myburgh KH, et al. Low bone mineral density at axial and appendicular sites in amenorrheic athletes. Med Sci Sports Exerc. 1993;25;1197.

2. BBC July 2006 Osteoporosis. Available from http://www.bbc.co.uk/health/conditions/osteoporosis1.shtml [cited 11 July 2007]

3. Cummings SR, et al. Endogenous hormones and the risk of hip and vertebral fractures among older women. N Engl J Med 1998;339:733.

4. LeBoff MS, et al. Occult vitamin D deficiency in postmenopausal US women with acute hip fracture. JAMA 1999;281:1505.

5. Thomas MK, et al. Hypovitaminosis D in medical inpatients. N Engl J Med 1998;338:784.

6. Bonjour J-P, et al. Critical years and stages of puberty for spinal and femoral bone mass accumulation during adolescence. J Clin Endocrinol Metab 1991;73:555.

7. Teegarden D, et al. Dietary calcium, protein and phosphorus are related to bone mineral density and content in young women. Am J Clin Nutr 1998;68:749.

8. Beck RB, and Shoemaker MR. Osteoporosis: Understanding key risk factors and therapeutic options. Phys Sportsmed 2000;28 (2):69.

9. Johnston CC Jr, et al. Calcium supplementation and increases in bone mineral density in children. N Engl J Med 1992;327:82.

10. Klesges RC, et al. Changes in bone mineral content in male athletes: mechanisms of action and intervention effects. JAMA 1996 1996;276:226.

11. Nieves JN, et al. Calcium potentiates the effect estrogen and calcitonin on bone mass: review and analysis. Am J Clin Nutr 1998;67:18.

12. American College of Sports Medicine. American College of Sports Medicine position stand on osteoporosis and exercise. Med Sci Sports Exerc 1995;27:I.

13. Bailey DA, et al. Growth, physical activity, and bone mineral acquisition. Exerc Sport Sci Rev 1996;24:233.

14. Boot AM, et al. Bone mineral density in children and adolescents: relation to puberty , calcium intake and physical activity. J Clin Endocrinal Metab 1997;82:57.

15. Cassell C, et al. Bone mineral density in elite 7-9-yr-old female gymnasts and swimmers. Med Sci Sports Exerc 1996;28:1243.

16. Kohrt WM, et al. HRT preserves increases in bone mineral density and reductions in body fat after a supervised exercise program. J Appl Physiol 1998;84:1506.

17. Nickols-Richardson SM, et al. Premenarcheal gymnasts possess higher bone mineral density than controls. Med Sci Sports Exerc, 2000;32:62.

18. Sinaki M, et al. A three year controlled, randomized trial of the effect of dose-specified loading and strengthening exercise on bone mineral density of spine and femur in non-athletic, physically active women. Bone 1996,19.233.

19. Ulrich CM, et al. Bone mineral density in mother-daughter pairs: relations to lifetime exercise, lifetime milk consumption, and calcium supplements. Am J Clin Nutr 1996;63:72.

20. Suominen H., Rahkila P. Bone mineral density of the calcaneus in 70- to 81-yr-old male athletes and a population sample. Med Sci Sports Exerc 1991;23:1227.

21. Ryan As, et al. Aerobic exercise maintains regional bone mineral density during weight loss in postmenopausal women. J Appl Physiol 1998;84:1305.

22. Alekel L, et al. Contributions of exercise, body composition, and age to bone mineral density in premenopausal women. Med Sci Sports Exerc 1995;27:1477.

23. Drinkwater BL. C.H. McCloy research lecture: does physical activity play a role in preventing osteoporosis? Res Q Exerc Sport 1994;65:197.

24. Dyson KC, et al. Gymnastics training and bone density in pre-adolescent

females. Med Sci Sports Exerc 1997;29:443.

25. Taaffe DR, et al. Differential effects of swimming versus weight bearing activity on bone mineral status of eumenorrheic athletes. J Bone Miner Res 1995;10:586.

26. Westerlind KC, et al. Effect of resistance exercise training on cortical and cancellous bone in mature male rats. J Appl Physiol 1998;84:459.

27. Robinson TL, et al. Gymnasts exhibit higher bone mass than runners despite similar prevalence of amenorrhea and oligomenorrhea. J Bone Miner Res 1995;10:26.

28. Layne JE, Nelson ME. The effects of progressive resistance training on bone density: a review. Med Sci Sports Exerc 1999;31:25.

WHY
EXERCISE?

**To Prevent or
Reduce Back Pain**

Why Exercise? - To Prevent or Reduce Back Pain

Understanding Back Pain

Back pain can range from a dull, constant ache to a sudden, sharp pain that leaves a person incapacitated. It can occur when someone lifts something that is too heavy or lifts something incorrectly. It can occur as the result of an accident or a fall. Often however, it develops slowly, as a result of age-related changes to the spine.

Regardless of how and why it happens, back pain can really diminish a person's quality of life. The lower back is under constant and continual stress from movements. However, the back can become much less vulnerable by strengthening it with regular exercise.

UK Statistics on Back Pain

Lower back pain is the most prevalent cause of disability in people under age 45. In the UK, lower back pain is one of the most common ailments. Studies show that approximately 60% to 80% of people living in Western societies experience back pain at some point in their life. Furthermore, experts are saying lower back pain is on the increase.

- Four in five adults will experience back pain. [1]

- About 80% of us will experience back pain over our lifetimes. [2]

- There are more than 8.5 million people in the UK who between them suffer from over 200 musculoskeletal conditions (MSCs). (Department of Health, 2004). [3]

- MSCs are the second most common cause of days off work in both men and women, with at an estimated cost to the economy of over 18 billion a year. (Arthritis Research Campaign, 2002). In 2002-3, 192 million days were lost to certified incapacity due to musculoskeletal conditions. (DWP Information and Analysis Directorate, 2004). [3]

- More than one in five GP visits involves the symptoms of a musculoskeletal condition. The main symptoms of MSCs include pain, stiffness, joint deformity, fatigue and impaired mobility. (Royal College of General Practitioners, 1996). [3]

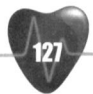

- More than 3 million people in the UK are affected by back pain that lasts more than one year. (A Maniadakis, A Gray, 2000). [3]

- MSCs are the leading cause of physical disability in the UK. (ARMA, 2004).

- 50% of people with arthritis say the worst aspect is pain. (Arthritis Research Campaign, 2002).

- The total cost of MSCs to health and social services in the UK is estimated as £5.5 billion a year. (Arthritis Research Campaign, 2002). [3]

- More than 39,000 hip and 39,000 knee replacements were performed in the UK in 2000. (Department of Health, 2004). [3]

- Around one in five claimants of incapacity benefit - nearly half a million people - have MSCs. **Payments of incapacity benefit to people with MSCs costs more than £30 million a week**. (DWP Information and Analysis Directorate, 2004). [3]

Symptoms of Back Pain

Pain in the back can come in several forms:

- Stiffness and pain when bending
- Pain accompanied by numbness and tingling
- Sharp pain felt in a specific area

Generally, it occurs as an aching pain in the lower back, which is eased and relieved by standing and made worse by sitting.

What does Back Pain generally lead to?

Back pain can lead to functional disability, numbness and weakness, chronic pain, sciatica, sleep problems and depression. Back pain can also signal nerve damage or other serious medical problems.

Why Does it Happen?

Experts believe that the major cause of lower back pain is sedentary lifestyles. Many people in industrialised countries are inactive both at work and home. People spend lots of time sitting in front of computers, driving in their cars, or glued to the couch, watching TV. As people sit, their backs are often not properly supported; this is bad for the spine. **Lower back pain is most certainly a lifestyle issue**.

Sports injuries often result in back problems later on in life. However, although the causes of back pain are usually physical, emotional stress can play a role in how severe the pain is, and how long it lasts.

Why Exercise?

Treating back pain with pain relief medication is really only a short-term "band aid" treatment for a chronic condition. For a long-term fix, the back muscles need to be strengthened. Regular exercise can accomplish this permanent solution.

Exercise is now recognised and accepted among the medical community as one of the essential ingredients of pain management. Strength and flexibility of the spine, along with cardiovascular fitness, may be the main benefits of regular exercise in general. For a distressed back to heal, it must be stimulated. Active back-pain exercises should be done in a controlled, gradual, and progressive manner. Movement of the back stimulates blood flow, which distributes nutrients into the disc space and soft tissues in the spine. This keeps the discs, muscles, ligaments and joints healthy, or restores health to the area. With a lack of movement, the back quickly becomes stiff, weak and deconditioned.

Remember when you were last confined to your bed by an illness? When you got up, did you feel relaxed and rejuvenated? Did you feel ready to tackle any task? Of course not, and illness wasn't the only cause. Bed rest and inactivity actually have a negative impact. Our bodies simply weren't designed to be stationary for too long.

The most common exercises to prevent and rehabilitate lower back pain are muscle-strengthening and joint-flexibility exercises. [4, 5, 6, 7] Furthermore, an active lifestyle aids rapid recovery from back pain. By isolating and strengthening the abdomen and lower back, muscles experience less pain and fewer chronic symptoms. This isolated conditioning also develops muscular strength, endurance, and range of motion. [8]

Maintaining a healthy weight also helps to minimise the risk of back pain. Healthy bodyweight will help maintain a healthy spine.

In Summary:

- As long as human beings walk upright we will always be susceptible to back pain, and its attendant difficulties. However, this natural tendency is greatly exacerbated by modern life which for most people is predominantly sedentary.

- Whatever your lifestyle habits and even if you already have a back problem, it makes good sense (under expert supervision) to provide your back with as much protection as possible. You can do this by a regular exercise programme that strengthens your back and abdominal muscles and increases vital circulation to the surrounding connective tissues.

Chapter References

1. BBC Back Pain. Available from http://www.bbc.co.uk/health/conditions/back_pain/ [cited 10 July 2007]

2. Health & Safety Executive 21 May 2007 Better Backs Campaign. Available from http://www.hse.gov.uk/msd/campaigns/getinvolved.htm [cited 10 July 2007]

3. Back Care Key facts about Musculoskeletal Conditions. Available from http://www.backpain.org/pages/a_pages/arma-mscs.php [cited 10 July 2007]

4. Bentsen H, et al. The effects of dynamic strength back exercise and/or home training program in 57-year-old women with chronic low back pain: results of a prospective randomized study with a 3-year follow-up period. Spine 1997;2:1494.

5. McGill SM. Low back stability: From frontal description to issues for performance and rehabilitation. Exerc Sport Sci Rev 2001;29:26;

6. Salminen JJ, et al.

7. Videman T, et al. Lumbar spinal pathology in cadaveric material in relation to history of back pain, occupation and physical loading. Spine 1990;15:728.

8. Carpenter DM, Nelson BW. Low back strengthening for the prevention and treatment of low back pain. Med Sci Sports Exerc 1999;31:18.

WHY
EXERCISE?

**To Prevent
Alzheimer's Disease**

Why Exercise? - To Prevent Alzheimer's Disease

Understanding Alzheimer's Disease

As people grow older, they can become increasingly forgetful, but severe loss of memory may be a sign of Alzheimer's Disease which is the most common cause of dementia. In this disorder, brain cells gradually degenerate and deposits of an abnormal protein build up in the brain. This build-up of protein causes brain tissue to shrink, which causes a progressive loss of mental abilities. The underlying cause of tissue destruction is presently unknown and as yet there is no cure for Alzheimer's Disease.

UK Statistics on Alzheimer's Disease

Current statistics show there are nearly 18 million people suffering with Alzheimer's Disease throughout the world.

There are over 100 different types of dementia. The most common is Alzheimer's Disease. [1]

- There are currently 700,000 people with dementia in the UK. [2]

- There are currently 15,000 younger people with dementia in the UK. [1]

- There are over 11,500 people with dementia from black and minority ethnic groups in the UK. [1]

- There will be over a million people with dementia by 2025. [1]

- Two thirds of people with dementia are women. [1]

- The proportion of people with dementia doubles for every 5 year age group. [1]

- One third of people over 95 have dementia. [1]

- 60,000 deaths a year are directly attributable to dementia. [1]

- Delaying the onset of dementia by 5 years would reduce deaths directly attributable to dementia by 30,000 a year. [1]

- The financial cost of dementia to the UK is over £17 billion a year. [1]

- Family carers of people with dementia save the UK over £6 billion

a year. [1]

- 64% of people living in care homes have a form of dementia. [1]
- Two thirds of people with dementia live in the community while one third live in a care home. [1]

Symptoms of Alzheimer's Disease

The first symptom of Alzheimer's Disease is usually forgetfulness. As we mentioned, there is a normal deterioration of memory as we age. But when this deterioration becomes severe, it affects intellectual ability. At this point, other symptoms usually appear.

Other symptoms of Alzheimer's Disease include:

- Difficulty in understanding written or spoken language
- Difficulty in general communication
- Poor concentration
- Becoming lost even in familiar surroundings

What does Alzheimer's Disease generally lead to?

As Alzheimer's Disease progresses, other symptoms appear. When people become aware they are losing their memory and becoming more forgetful, depression and anxiety can occur.

Severe symptoms of Alzheimer's Disease are:

- Rapid mood swings
- Severe personality changes (e.g. aggression)
- Unsteadiness walking and moving in general

Why Does it Happen?

Scientists are not yet sure what causes Alzheimer's Disease. There are probably several factors that affect each person differently. Age is the most important known factor for Alzheimer's, as the number of people with the disease doubles every 5 years beyond age 65.

Scientists still need to learn a lot more about what causes Alzheimer's Disease. In addition to genetics, they are also studying movement, exercise, education, diet and environment to learn what role they play in the development of this disease.

Why Exercise?

Scientific Research on Alzheimer's Disease & Exercise

A study published in the Journal of the American Medical Association involving 18,766 women between 70 and 81 years of age, found that just walking approximately half a kilometre each day reduced dementia by 20 - 50%. The lead author, Dr. Jennifer Weuve of the Harvard School of Public Health in Boston said, "We were a bit surprised that walking would be associated with cognitive benefits."

Another study, also published in the Journal of the American Medical Association involving 2,257 men between 71 and 93 years of age revealed that men who walked less than 500 metres each day had an 80% greater risk of developing dementia than men who walked three kilometres or more daily. The author was Dr. Robert Abbott, a Biostatistician at the University of Virginia in Charlottesville, VA. Abbott stressed that while exercise clearly benefits the mind and the body, a lifetime of active behaviour and exercise is really needed. Dr. Abbott went on to say that people who are active and adhere to a healthier lifestyle and better diet will benefit by overall long-term health of the brain.

Dr. Robert Friedland, Associate Professor of Neurology, Psychiatry and Radiology at Case Western Reserve University in Cleveland, conducted some pertinent research. Friedland talked about his findings at the annual meeting of the American Academy of Neurology. He said, "People who were less active in their leisure time activities were three to four times more likely to develop Alzheimer's disease as compared with those who were more active away from work."

In previous studies, Friedland and his colleagues showed that physical activity seemed to work as a preventative measure against Alzheimer's Disease. His studies have involved family members to accurately profile patients' leisure activities, as Alzheimer's patients have severe memory loss and could not reliably report their actions to document a professional research study.

Carl Cotman, Director of the Institute for Brain Aging and Dementia at UC Irvine's College of Medicine, and Nicole Berchtold, a researcher at the same institute, conducted another study. Their findings were

published in Trends in Neurosciences. Cotman and Berchtold reported that **a daily jog might prevent the deterioration of brain cells that can lead to Alzheimer's Disease**. Cotman and Berchtold explained that scientists have only recently started to look at exercise as a possible preventative measure against Alzheimer's Disease. In their study with rats, they found that exercise is a powerful regulator of brain activity.

Between 1992 and 2000, Constantine G. Lyketsos, M.D., Professor of Psychiatry and Behavioral Sciences at Johns Hopkins, studied 3,375 65-year-old men and women. His subjects did not have dementia at the start of the study. The concluding data, published in Journal Cell, showed clearly that **dementia occurred significantly less frequently in those who exercised and lived active lives. Lyketsos said, "Exercise works to reduce the risk of dementia**."

A very unique study was conducted by Drs. Kevin M. Guskiewiez, Professor of Exercise and Sport Science in the UNC College of Arts and Sciences, and Stephen W. Marshall, Associate Professor of Epidemiology at the UNC School of Public Health and of Orthopedics at the UNC School of Medicine. Guskiewiez and Marshall showed that recurrent concussions and sub-concussive contact to the head may be linked to an early expression of Alzheimer's Disease.

This study surveyed 3,683 retired professional football players who belonged to the NFL Retired Players' Association. The players were asked if there had been any long-term consequences from concussions or 'head contact' while playing in the NFL. Many retired players reported that previous concussions and head contact had a permanent effect on their thinking and memory skills as they aged. Also, in this study, retired players who had experienced three or more concussions had a five-fold greater chance of being diagnosed with Alzheimer's.

Researchers from the U.S. National Institute on Aging (NIA) and Duke University in North Carolina have found that head injuries are related to Alzheimer's Disease. They found that a head injury in childhood or early adult life is associated with an increased risk for Alzheimer's and dementia later on. The study, published in the Journal of Neurology, also found that the severity of head injury increased the risk of Alzheimer's.

In Summary:

- Alzheimer's Disease, or any other type of dementia, is usually age-related and therefore increasingly prevalent with the rise in general life expectancy.

- Whilst there are no absolute guarantees, it is quite clear that - as with any disease predominantly linked to the process of ageing – developing a lifelong habit of regular exercise will significantly increase one's chances of delaying, or even completely avoiding, such problems.

Chapter References

1. Alzheimer's Society Facts about dementia. Available from: http://www.alzheimers.org.uk/Facts_about_dementia/Statistics/index.htm [cited 9 July 2007]

2. Allender, S., Peto, V., Scarborough, P., Boxer, A., Rayner, M. (2006) Coronary Heart Disease Statistics. British Heart Foundation, London.

WHY
EXERCISE?

To Prevent
Parkinson's Disease

Why Exercise? - To Prevent Parkinson's Disease

Understanding Parkinson's Disease

Parkinson's Disease tends to manifest itself after the age of 60 and is more common in men than women. The disease results from a degeneration of nerve cells in the basal ganglia. The basal ganglia controls the smoothness of muscle movements. Thus, Parkinson's is characterised by shaking or tremors, difficulty walking, stiff movement and lack of coordination.

These muscular problems are caused by nerve cell degeneration. Cells in the affected part of the brain are responsible for producing dopamine. Parkinson's causes these cells to degenerate and decrease in number, which causes a decrease in dopamine. Reduced dopamine causes an imbalance with acetylcholine. The result is the characteristic stiff, disjointed and uncoordinated movement described above.

UK Statistics on Parkinson's Disease

Parkinson's Disease is among the most prevalent neurological disorders; globally at least four million people have it. Each year, there are as many as 50,000 new cases being diagnosed worldwide.

- The Parkinson's Disease Society estimates there are about 120,000 people in the UK with the disease - that's one in 500 of the general population - and approximately 10,000 new cases are diagnosed each year. [1]

- Parkinson's is a progressive neurological condition that's usually diagnosed after the age of 60, although one in 20 people diagnosed will be under 40 at the time of diagnosis. [1]

Generally, in the UK:

- 1 in 500 people, around 120,000 individuals, have Parkinson's

- about 10,000 people in the UK are diagnosed each year

- symptoms first appear, on average, when a patient is older than 50

- 1 in 20 of those diagnosed each year will be aged under 40 years

- statistically, men are slightly more likely to develop Parkinson's

than women. [2]

Symptoms of Parkinson's Disease

Parkinson's Disease is progressive, which means symptoms get worse over time. Initial symptoms are very subtle, such as a slight tremor or shaking of the hand. At first, moving the hand may make the shaking temporarily subside. However, later on, tremors usually affect the other hand and other parts of the body to include: arms, legs and the head, jaw and tongue. With stress, tremors usually increase.

As the disease progresses, movement becomes difficult and muscles stiffen, which makes movement jerky and awkward. Sufferers can sometimes freeze in the middle of a movement. Parkinson's sufferers often have difficulty speaking, writing, and with movement in general.

Parkinson's Disease sufferers often look expressionless, as though they feel no emotion. This occurs as facial muscles become very rigid. Other symptoms often include: a speech problem, sleep disorders, abdominal cramps, constipation and an inability to urinate.

What does Parkinson's Disease generally lead to?

Parkinson's Disease often leads to dementia and depression. Sufferers usually experience a progressive loss of intellectual function and a loss of awareness of reality.

Why Does it Happen?

The cause of Parkinson's Disease is unknown. Recent scientific studies on twins suggest that genetic factors may not play much of a role. Studies suggest a link to possible environmental factors, such as emotional stress, poor diet and a lack of physical exercise. These factors increase the risk of developing Parkinson's Disease.

Why Exercise?

Scientific Research on Parkinson's Disease & Exercise

William Weiner, M.D., of the University of Maryland School of Medicine in Baltimore spoke at the American Academy of Neurology's 58th annual meeting. Weiner said, "**There are no drugs that can prevent or turn back Parkinson's Disease: there are none**." He went on to say, "**About the only**

steps that appear to have any value are exercise and physical therapy."

Scientists from the McKnight Brain Institute of the University of Florida conducted a study on the effects of exercise on the brain. They showed that lifelong exercise decreases cellular ageing in the brain. Their study on rats revealed that moderately active rats have healthier DNA and more robust brain cells than less active rats. Thomas Foster, Ph.D., Chairman of the McKnight Brain Institute for Brain Research in Memory Loss at the College of Medicine, said, "The results show **regular, mild exercise can prevent oxidative damage in the brain**." Oxidative damage has been associated with Alzheimer's Disease and Parkinson's Disease. It occurs as a natural consequence of ageing and is a contributing factor to memory loss.

Eric Klann, Ph.D., Professor of Molecular Physiology and Biophysics at the Baylor College of Medicine was not connected to the research, but reviewed the work. Klann said, "The difference between humans and rats is that it isn't easy to get humans to exercise."

Dr. Jeff Bronstein, a Parkinson's expert says, "Exercise definitely works and plays a role in the treatment of Parkinson's Disease." He continues, "Physiologically, it retrains the brain. Automatic or implicit memory functions – things you do without thinking – get reinforced through exercise. There is some evidence that neurons are actually regenerated."

In Summary:

- **Parkinson's Disease is usually a problem that manifests itself in later life. Once diagnosed, there is little that contemporary medicine can offer apart from palliative treatments.**

- **However, as recent research indicates that Parkinson's Disease, like so many other conditions, is symptomatic of physical neglect, the best thing we can do to reduce the risk is to strengthen the immune system by committing to a good exercise programme.**

Chapter References

1. BBC January 2007 Parkinson's Disease. Available from http://www.bbc.co.uk/health/conditions/parkinsons1.shtml [cited 11 July 2007[

2. Parkinson's Disease Society How Many People Have Parkinson's? Available from http://www.parkinsons.org.uk/about-parkinsons/what-is-parkinsons/how-many-people-have-parkinson.aspx [cited July 11 2007]

WHY EXERCISE?

To Prevent
Multiple Sclerosis

Why Exercise? - To Prevent Multiple Sclerosis

Understanding Multiple Sclerosis

MS is an autoimmune disorder in which the body's immune system attacks its own nervous system tissues, resulting in the progressive damage of nerves in the brain and spinal cord.

Nerves are covered by myelin, which acts as a protective insulating sheath. However, with MS, small areas of myelin become damaged. This is known as demyelination. When myelin is damaged, the nerves become inflamed and impulses cannot be carried effectively along nerves.

Generally there are two types of MS:

• Relapse-remitting MS (RRMS)

• Chronic-progressive MS (CPMS)

In RRMS, symptoms usually last for a few days and then clear up. Symptoms may reappear at any time, and often with progressively worsening effects. In some cases, a person with RRMS may eventually develop CPMS.

With CPMS, there is a gradual, progressive worsening of symptoms and deterioration.

UK Statistics on Multiple Sclerosis

• MS is the most common neurological disorder among young adults, affecting 85,000 people in the UK, with 2,500 newly diagnosed each year. It's more common in temperate rather than tropical climates. Scotland has the highest incidence in the world. Onset is usually between 20 and 40 years of age. [1]

• It is the most common disabling neurological condition affecting young adults. Around 85,000 people in the UK have MS. [2]

• It's more common in women, with a ratio of two men to three women affected. [2] It strikes most often during early adulthood.

• **Over time, more women are developing MS than men**, according to research that was presented at the American Academy of Neurology's 59th Annual Meeting in Boston, April 28 – May 5,

2007. [3]

- In 1940, the ratio of women to men with MS in the United States was approximately two to one. By 2000, that ratio had grown to approximately four to one. [3]

- "That's an increase in the ratio of women to men of nearly 50 percent per decade," said study author Gary Cutter, PhD, of the University of Alabama at Birmingham School of Public Health. "We don't yet know why more women are developing MS than men, and more research is needed." [3]

- Cutter said researchers will need to explore multiple changes that have occurred for women over the last several decades, including the use of oral contraceptives, earlier menstruation, obesity rates, changes in smoking rates, and later age of first births. [3]

Symptoms of Multiple Sclerosis

Multiple sclerosis symptoms can vary immensely, because MS can affect many sites in the nervous system.

Common symptoms include:

- Numbness or tingling in any part of the body

- Tiredness/fatigue

- Blurred vision

- Weakness and heaviness in the arms and legs

- Problems with balance and coordination

What does Multiple Sclerosis generally lead to?

MS can lead to depression, memory lapses, muscle weakness and painful muscle spasms. Eventually, damage to myelin may cause paralysis and severely affected individuals may need wheelchairs.

Why Does it Happen?

The cause of MS is unknown. However genetics, immune responses and environmental factors are the most likely culprits. It has been postulated that an environmental factor during childhood might play an important role in the development of MS later in life. However, no conclusive evidence has been found for any particular environmental factor.

Why Exercise?

Scientific Research on Multiple Sclerosis & Exercise

Dr. Walter R. Frontera, Chairman of Harvard Medical School Department of Physical Medicine and Rehabilitation and Director of the Muscle Cell Physiology Laboratory at Spaulding Rehabilitation Hospital, says that exercise can be useful when Multiple Sclerosis is more stable. He recommends exercises to maintain or increase flexibility, muscle strength and cardiovascular endurance.

Dr. Barry Oken, Neurologist at Oregon Health and Science University, published a study in the Journal Neurology. Oken found that stretching exercises are an effective form of treatment for MS sufferers. This study showed that MS patients who stretched regularly had significantly less fatigue than those who didn't.

Aerobic exercise is also thought to help people with MS fight fatigue, the most common symptom of the disease. Nadine Fisher, Ed.D. is Clinical Associate Professor of Rehabilitation Science in the UB School of Public Health and Health Professions. After a study on MS and exercise, Fisher said, "Exercise is good for MS, it can build up strength and endurance, reduce depression and increase endorphins, the chemicals in the brain responsible for positive moods, but it must be done correctly."

A study on MS patients done at the Wright State University School of Medicine, Dayton, OH, showed that exercise training can improve both cardiorespiratory fitness and skeletal muscle function for MS patients.

Dr. Bernadette Kalman, Director of MS Research at St. Luke's – Roosevelt Hospital Center, Columbia University and Assistant Professor of Neurology, Columbia University also commented on the effects of exercise. Kalman says that inactive muscles atrophy over time, which can further increase motor disability. **Exercise can prevent muscle and cell atrophy**, and improve motor skills. Regular exercise is very beneficial both physically and mentally to prevent and treat MS.

Dr. Tomas Olsson, Director of the Department of Molecular Medicine, at Karolinska Institute in Stockholm, Sweden, says that there are many good studies on the benefits of exercise and MS and he recommends exercise to all MS patients.

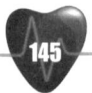

In another study in the Journal of Neurology, fifty-four MS patients were randomly assigned to non-exercise and exercise groups. The exercise group demonstrated significant increases in VO2 max. VO2 max is the maximum amount of oxygen (in millilitres) that an individual can use in one minute per kilogram of body weight. It is a scientific measure of cardiovascular fitness. The exercise group also showed improvement in upper and lower extremity strength. In addition, depression and anger scores were significantly reduced and they showed significant improvements for social interaction, emotional behaviour, home management, recreation, and pastimes. Exercise training resulted in improved fitness and had a positive impact on factors related to quality of life.

Dr. Adam Kaplin, Chief Psychiatric Consultant to the MS Centre at Johns Hopkins University School of Medicine, says that regular exercise is very important as a treatment for MS sufferers. It maximises independence and stimulates the central nervous system (CNS). Exercise can actually work to repair damage to the CNS by activating neighbouring pathways in the brain.

Finally, Dr. Werner is Professor of Neurology at Harvard Medical School and Director of the MS Centre in the Brigham and Women's Hospital in Massachusetts General Hospital. Werner says that **exercise is extremely important for the nervous system to remain healthy**.

In Summary:

- **No question, Multiple Sclerosis occurs when the autoimmune system malfunctions, so an effective exercise programme that contains an aerobic element and stretching movements to improve circulation is the best way to increase your defences against this frightening disease.**

- **Furthermore, research clearly confirms that such measures are equally useful to reduce the severity of the symptoms in existing MS sufferers.**

Chapter References
1. BBC July 2006 Multiple Sclerosis. Available from http://www.bbc.co.uk/health/conditions/ms1.shtml [cited 11 July 2007]

2. Multiple Sclerosis Society 1 June 2007 About MS. Available from http://www.mssociety.org.uk/about_ms/index.html {cited 11 July 2007]

3. The Multiple Sclerosis Resource Centre   Gender and MS. Available from http://www.msrc.co.uk/index.cfm?fuseaction=show&pageid=1855   [cited 11 July 2007]

17

WHY
EXERCISE?

To Ensure Optimum
Health & Longevity

Why Exercise? - To Ensure Optimum Health & Longevity

Chronic disease prevention, treatment and healthcare help people to live longer, happier and more productive lives. [1]

As a species, humans in this century and the last have failed to adapt to sedentary lifestyles, smoking, alcohol and stress. [2, 3] Lack of physical activity causes nearly 30% of all deaths from heart disease, diabetes and colon cancer. [4] However, physical exercise can significantly reduce mortality from degenerative diseases in older adults and greatly improve cardiovascular function, muscle strength and quality of life. [5, 6, 7] Physical exercise at any age helps to extend life. [8, 9] Statistics show that people who adopt healthier lifestyles live longer and postpone and diminish their level of disability toward the end of life. [10]

Health span could be described as the total number of years an individual remains in good health. There is little point in living longer if the added years are unhealthy, unproductive, unhappy and painful.

Successful ageing requires ongoing physical exercise and maintenance. Research and statistics now view ageing in general as lifestyle-related. Physical and mental deterioration is dependent on lifestyle and environmental influences: primarily improper diet and lack of exercise. [9, 11, 12] With better lifestyle habits, including exercise, people can avoid many health problems.

Among other benefits, good lifestyle habits can improve:

• Preservation of muscular strength

• Maintenance of joint range-of-motion

• Quality of sleep

• Cardiovascular function [6, 13, 14, 15, 16]

Life expectancy has been used for many years to estimate overall length of life. However, it does little to establish quality of life, especially as age progresses. Healthy life expectancy was introduced in 2000 by the World Health Organization (WHO) (www.who.int/whr) to establish the expected number of years that a person may live in full health.

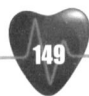

Research suggests that possibly less than 10% of adults in the US, England, Australia and Canada exercise with enough intensity to receive discernable health benefits. In addition, adult and adolescent females participate in lower levels of regular physical exercise than adult or adolescent men. [17]

It is possible that the decrease in physical activity, as humans age, has a biological basis. Current debates suggest that dopamine production (which regulates motivation for movement) decreases as we age. [18] Physical inactivity results in an array of degenerative problems and conditions that eventually lead to premature death. Sedentary death syndrome (SEDS) is a term now being used to describe this condition. [19]

Chronic degenerative diseases in adults have increased dramatically worldwide due to poor diet and physical inactivity. Even children are now developing SEDS-related diseases, which include:

• Obesity

• Atherosclerosis

• Cardiovascular disease

It is estimated that SEDS will cost the US alone $2-3 trillion in healthcare expenses in the next 10 years.

Research shows functional physiologic capacity improves to approximately age 30, and then naturally declines with age. Although the number of long-term exercise studies are limited, research has shown a 50-year-old who participates in regular physical exercise often maintains the functional level of a 20-year-old. Exercise overrides the deterioration in physiologic function that usually occurs with ageing. [20, 21, 22] Accelerated muscular strength loss coincides with the increase of many chronic diseases, such as:

• Arthritis

• Stroke

• Diabetes

• Coronary heart disease [23]

In addition, loss of muscular strength in the elderly directly relates to poor balance, fatigue and weakness. These factors lead to an increased incidence of accidents. [24]

Moderate resistance training can be a safe way to slow deteriorating muscular strength and diminishing muscle mass that accompanies the ageing process. [25, 26, 27, 28] **Studies now show that muscle responds to training with improved strength adaptations, even into the ninth decade of life**. [29] Regular exercise is an effective means to improve muscle strength, bone density, balance and more. It is also specifically a way to avoid the physical frailty that is normally associated with ageing. [30]

A physically active life positively affects neuromuscular functions that normally slow in age. Typically, these functions diminish in relation to performance of cognitive processing. [31] However, **elderly individuals who remain active show information processing reaction speeds that equal or exceed inactive individuals in their 20s!** [32]

Research indicates that age typically causes a decline in VO2 max (the maximum amount of oxygen an individual can use in one minute per kilogram of body weight). This decline is nearly twice as fast in sedentary men and women as those who exercise regularly throughout life. In fact, **living a sedentary life causes a loss in functional cardiovascular capacity at least as great as the effects of ageing**.

Older individuals sustain a high degree of trainability often equal to younger individuals and can benefit positively from muscular and cardiovascular adaptations. [33, 34] Elderly men can increase aerobic capacity to the same relative extent (15 to 30%) as younger adults. [30, 35, 36, 37]

Regular weight-bearing exercise increases bone mass in elderly men and women. [38] In postmenopausal women, regular exercise augments hormone replacement therapy and helps to prevent osteoporosis. [39]

Elderly individuals experience increased levels of disease prevalence largely due to increased body fat in the abdominal region, which is caused by poor diet and inadequate physical activity. [40]

Research concludes that exercise training improves physiologic function at any age. Several factors contribute to the magnitude of change experienced.

These factors include:

• Genetics

• Initial fitness level

• Specific type of exercise training

In research studies, exercise often causes overall health to improve – as a result of physiologic adaptation – whatever a person's age. [41, 42]

For some time, studies have been showing that exercise lengthens lifespan. [43] One of the first studies showed that former Harvard oarsmen had lengthened their predicted lifespan by 5.1 years. [44] However, studies suggest that athletic participation as an adolescent and young adult does <u>not</u> ensure health and longevity later on in life. [45] **Analysis of much research is concluding that exercise needs to be maintained throughout life to provide significant health and longevity benefits**. [46, 47, 48, 49, 50]

A study of 17,000 Harvard alumni who attended college between 1916 and 1950 provided significant evidence that those who performed moderate aerobic exercise added several years to their life. In contrast, those who exercised to the extreme (marathons, sports competitions, etc.) had higher death rates than those who exercised moderately or those who were inactive. [51]

This research provided significant evidence that moderate exercise is best to extend life. [52] Active men live the longest, largely due to reduced death from cardiovascular disease. Indeed, **it is estimated that the risk associated with living a sedentary lifestyle and not exercising, is equal to the risk of smoking one pack of cigarettes a day!**

An analysis of 43 studies on the relationship between physical inactivity and cardiovascular disease concluded that a lack of exercise promotes cardiovascular disease in a cause-and-effect manner. [53, 54, 55]

Fitness alone is a strong independent predictor of disease and all-cause mortality. [56, 57, 58] **Moderate-intensity regular exercise significantly reduces the risk of heart disease, cancer and early death**. [59, 60, 29] **Studies show conclusively that regular exercise protects against heart disease**. [61, 62, 63, 64] Independent of physical activity (such as gardening and active work), aerobic exercise provides significant protection against the risk factors and occurrence of cardiovascular disease. [65, 66]

In Summary:

- **Use it, … or lose it!**

- **A gradual loss of physical ability is of course a natural consequence of the ageing process, however well we try to look after ourselves.**

- **Now the good news: there is absolutely no doubt that, if we exercise sensibly, and consistently, throughout our lives we can remain fit and healthy for far longer than was previously thought possible. Indeed, regular physical exercise is an important ingredient in developing, and maintaining, quality of life – at any age!**

Chapter References

1. Frisoni GB, et al. Longevity and the epsilon2 allele of apolipoprotein E: the Finnish Centenarians Study. J Gerontol A Biol Sci Med Sci 2001;56:M75.

2. Visser M, et al. High body fatness, but not low fat-free mass, predicts disability in older men and women: the Cardiovascular Health Study. Am J Clin Nutr 1998;68:584.

3. Vita AJ, et al. Aging, health risks, and cumulative disability. N Engl J Med 1998;338:1035.

4. Martinez ME, et al. Physical activity, body mass index, and prostaglandin E2 levels in rectal mucosa. J Natl Cancer Inst 1999;91:950.

5. Bronstrup A, et al. Effects of folic acid and combinations of folic acid and vitamin B-12 on plasma homocysteine concentrations in healthy young women. Am J Clin Nutr 1998;68:1104.

6. Huang Y, et al. Physical fitness, physical activity, and functional limitation in adults aged 40 and older. Med Sci Sports Exerc 1998;30:1430.

7. Kosta T, et al. Habitual physical activity and peak anaerobic power in elderly women. Eur J Appl Physiol 1997;76:81.

8. Paffenbarger RS Jr, et al. Changes in physical activity and other life-way patterns influencing longevity. Med Sci Sports Exerc 1994;26:857.

9. Stampfer MJ, et al. Primary prevention of coronary heart disease in women through diet and lifestyle. N Engl J Med 2000;343:92.

10. Powell KE, Blair SN. The public health burdens of sedentary living habits: theoretical but realistic estimates. Med Sci Sports Exerc 1994;26:851.

11. Finch EE, Tanzi RE, Genetics of aging. Science 1997;278:407.

12. Lamberts SWJ, et al. The endocrinology of aging. Science 1997;278:419.

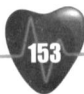

13. Brill PA, et al. Muscular strength and physical function. Med Sci Sports Exerc 2000;32:412.

14. Morey MC, et al. Is there a threshold between peak oxygen uptake and self-reported physical functioning in older adults? Med Sci Sports Exerc 1998;30:1223.

15. Morey MC, et al. Physical fitness and functional limitations in community-dwelling older adults. Med Sci Sports Exerc 1998;30:715

16. Sherrill DL, et al. Association of physical activity and human sleep disorders. Arch Intern Med 1998;158:1894.

17. Caspersen CJ, et al. Changes in physical activity patterns in the United States, by sex and cross-sectional age. Med Sci Sports Exerc 2000;32:1601.

18. Ingram DK. Age-related decline in physical activity: generalization to nonhumans. Med Sci Sports Exerc 2000;32:1623.

19. Booth FW, et al. Waging war on modern chronic diseases: primary prevention through exercise biology. J Appl Physiol 2000;88:774.

20. Hagerman FC, et al. A 20-year longitudinal study of Olympic oarsmen. Med Sci Sports Exerc 1996;28:1150.

21. Pollack ML, et al. Twenty-year follow-up of aerobic power and body composition of older track athletes. J Appl Physiol 1997;82:1508

22. Seiler KS, et al. Gender differences in rowing performance and power with aging. Med Sci Sports Exerc 1998;30:121.

23. Rantanken T, et al. Grip strength changes over 27 year in Japanese-American men. J Appl Physiol 1998;85:2047.

24. Johnston RB, et al. Effect of lower extremity muscular fatigue on motor control performance. Med Sci Sports Exerc 1998;30:1703.

25. ACSM position stand on exercise and physical activity for older adults. Med Sci Sports Exerc 1998;30:992.

26. McCartney N. Acute responses to resistance training and safety. Med Sci Sports Exerc 1999;31:31.

27. Pollack ML, et al. The recommended quantity and quality of exercise for developing and maintaining cardiorespiratory fitness, strength, and flexibility in healthy adults. Med Sci Sports Exerc 1998;30:975.

28. Tracy BL, et al. Muscle quality. II. Effects of strength training in 65 to 75-year-old men and women. J Appl Physiol 1999;86:195.

29. Wannamethee SG, et al. Changes in physical activity, mortality, and incidence of coronary heart disease in older men. Lancet 1998;351.

30. Bouvier F, et al. Left ventricular function and perfusion in elderly endurance athletes. Med Sci Sports Exerc 2001;33:735.

31. Van Boxtel MPJ, et al. Aerobic capacity and cognitive performance in a cross-sectional aging study. Med Sci Sports Exerc 1997;29:1357.

32. Spirduso WW, Clifford, P. Replication of age and physical activity effects on reaction and movement time. J Gerontol 1978;33:26.

33. Cartee GD. Influence of age on skeletal muscle glucose transport and glycogen metabolism. Med Sci Sports Exerc 1994;26:577.

34. Straton JR, et al. Cardiovascular responses to exercise: effects of aging. Circulation 1994;89:1648.

35. Ehsani AA, et al. Exercise training improves left ventricular systolic function in older men. Circulation 1991;83:96.

36. Levy WC, et al. Endurance exercise training augments diastolic filling at rest and during exercise in healthy young and older men. Circulation 1993;88:116.

37. Seals DR, et al. Enhanced left ventricular performance in endurance trained older men. Circulation 1994;89:198.

38. Layne JE, Nelson ME. The effects of progressive resistance training on bone density: a review. Med Sci Sports Exerc 1999;31:25.

39. Kohrt WM, et al. HRT preserves increases in bone mineral density and reductions in body fat after a supervised exercise program. J Appl Physiol 1998;84:1506.

40. ACSM position stand on exercise and type 2 diabetes. Med Sci Sports Exerc 2000;32:1345.

41. Cartee GD. Aging skeletal muscle: response to exercise. Exerc Sport Sci Rev 1994;22:91.

42. Coggan AR, et al. Skeletal muscle adaptations to endurance training in 60- to 70-year-old men and women. J Appl Physiol 1992;72:1780.

43. Andersen WG. Further studies on the longevity of Yale athletes. Med Times 1916;44:75.

44. Hill AB. Cricket and its relation to the duration of life. Lancet 1927;2:949.

45. Quinn TJ, et al. Caloric expenditure, life status, and disease in former male athletes and non-athletes. Med Sci Sports Exerc 1990;22:742.

46. Blair SN, et al. Changes in physical fitness and all cause mortality: a prospective study of healthy and unhealthy men. JAMA 1995;273:1093.

47. Blair SN, et al. Influences of cardiovascular fitness and other precursors on cardiovascular disease and all-cause mortality in men and women. JAMA 1996;276:205.

48. Farrell SW, et al. Influence of cardiorespiratory fitness levels and other predictors on cardiovascular disease mortality in men. Med Sci Sports Exerc 1998;30:899.

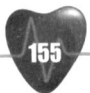

49. Heim DL, et al. Exercise mitigates the association of abdominal obesity with high-density lipoprotein cholesterol in premenopausal women: results from the third National Health and Nutrition Examination survey. J Am Diet Assoc 2000;100:1347.

50. Sandvik L, et al. Physical fitness as a predictor of mortality among healthy, middle-aged Norwegian men. N Engl J Med 1993;328:533.

51. Paffenbarger RS Jr, et al. Physical activity, all-cause mortality, and longevity of college alumni. N Engl J Med 1986;314:605.

52. Lee I-M, Paffenbarger RS. Exercise intensity and longevity in men: the Harvard Alumni study. JAMA 1995;273:1179.

53. Powell KE, et al. Physical activity and the incidence of coronary heart disease. Annu Rev Public Health 1987;8:253.

54. Farrell SW, et al. Influence of cardiorespiratory fitness levels and other predictors on cardiovascular disease mortality in men. Med Sci Sports Exerc 1998;30:899.

55. McMurray RG, et al. Is physical activity or aerobic power more influential on reducing cardiovascular disease risk factors? Med Sci Sports Exerc 1998;30:1521.

56. Williams PT. Physical fitness and activity as separate heart disease risk factors: a meta-analysis. Exer Sport Sci Rev 2001;33:754.

57. Dvorak RV, et al. Respiratory fitness, free living physical activity, and cardiovascular disease risk in older individuals: a doubly labeled water study. J Clin Endocrinol Metab 2000;85:957.

58. Wei M, et al. Relationship between low cardiorespiratory fitness and mortality in normal-weight, overweight, and obese men. JAMA 1999;282:1547.

59. Casazza GA, et al. Exercise training and reduction in some coronary risk factors in female cigarette smokers. Am J Cardiol 1995;75:85.

60. Kavanagh TT. Exercise in the primary prevention of coronary artery disease. Can J Cardiol 2001;17(2):155.

61. Blair SN. Physical activity, physical fitness, and health. Res Q Exec Sport 1993;64:365.

62. Morris JN. Exercise in the prevention of coronary heart disease: today's best bet in public health. Med Sci Sports Exerc 1994;26:807.

63. Pate RR, et al. Physical activity and public health: a recommendation from the Centers for Disease Control and Prevention and American College of Sports Medicine. JAMA 1995;273:402.

64. Thune I, et al. Physical activity improves the metabolic risk profile in men and women. Arch Intern Med 1998;158:1633.

65. Abbott RF, et al. Cardiovascular risk factors and graded treadmill exercise

endurance in healthy adults: the Framingham offspring Study. Am J Cardiol 1989:63:342.

66. Heim DL, et al. Exercise mitigates the association of abdominal obesity with high-density lipoprotein cholestrol in premenopausal women: results from the third National Health and Nutrition Examination survey. J Am Diet Assoc 2000:100:1347.

WHY EXERCISE?

EXERCISE?

**To Positively
Influence Children**

Why Exercise - To Positively Influence Children

I hope this book has helped you to become more aware of the value of exercise, and that it will motivate you to take more responsibility for your health than ever before.

Today, in 2007, more adults desperately need to start exercising regularly so that children and adolescents are positively influenced by their behaviour.

Studies have shown that atherosclerosis (and therefore, cardiovascular disease) can develop even during adolescence. [1] **Autopsies of young children have revealed that fatty streaks and plaque in coronary arteries appear even in the very young**. [2] However, when children participate in exercise early on, the risk of atherosclerosis may be reduced even later in life. [3, 4] Children need to be taught in school about the risk factors involved with sedentary lifestyles. They should also be taught, at school and at home, about the benefits of exercising regularly. [5]

The European Heart Study has recently revealed that the clogging of arteries starts in early life. This study checked 1,700 children between 9 and 15. Dr. Ekelund, of the Medical Research Council epidemiology unit in Cambridge declared after this study that "It is clear that low levels of physical activity in children is associated with risk factors that are known to increase the risk factors of cardiovascular disease in later life."

The current UK guidelines recommend children need an hour of exercise daily, but studies are suggesting that only one in 10 children are achieving this goal. If you are a parent, try to work with your local school to change this and encourage your friends to exercise more frequently too. Pass this book on to a friend, or your local school. Aim to positively influence those around you, especially the young, to exercise more.

Wholeheartedly

Anthony Aurelius

Chapter References

1. Strong JP, et al. Prevalence and extent of atherosclerosis in adolescents and young adults. JAMA 1999,281:727.

2. Berenson GS, et al. Association between multiple cardiovascular risk factors and atherosclerosis in children and young adults. N Engl J Med 1998;338:1650.

3. Depres J-P, et al. Physical activity and coronary heart disease risk factors during childhood and adolescence. Exerc Sport Sci Rev 1990;18.

4. Williams PT. Physical fitness and activity as separate heart disease risk factors: a meta-analysis. Exerc Sport Sci Rev 2001;33:754.

5. Killen JD, et al. Cardiovascular disease risk reduction for tenth graders. A multiple-factor school-based program. JAMA 1988;260:1728.